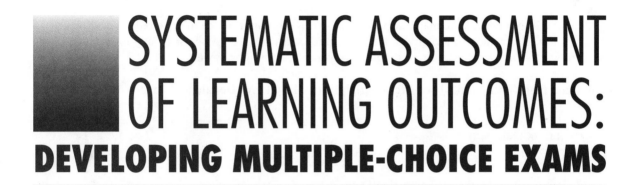

SYSTEMATIC ASSESSMENT OF LEARNING OUTCOMES:
DEVELOPING MULTIPLE-CHOICE EXAMS

Mary E. McDonald

JONES AND BARTLETT PUBLISHERS
Sudbury, Massachusetts
BOSTON   TORONTO   LONDON   SINGAPORE

World Headquarters
Jones and Bartlett Publishers
40 Tall Pine Drive
Sudbury, MA 01776
978-443-5000
info@jbpub.com
www.jbpub.com

Jones and Bartlett Publishers Canada
6339 Ormindale Way
Mississauga, ON L5V 1J2
CANADA

Jones and Bartlett Publishers International
Barb House, Barb Mews
London W6 7PA
UK

ISBN-13: 978-0-7637-1174-0
ISBN-10: 0-7637-1174-8

Library of Congress Cataloging-in-Publication Data

McDonald, Mary E.
    Systematic assessment of learning outcomes: developing multiple-choice exams / Mary E. McDonald.
        p. cm.
    Includes bibliographical references and index.
    ISBN 0-7637-1174-8
    1. Multiple-choice examinations. 2. Examinations—Design and construction. 3. Nursing—Examinations—Design and construction. I. Title.

    LB3060.32.M85 M33 2001
    371.26'1—dc21

2001029737

6048

Production Credits
Acquisitions Editor: Penny M. Glynn
Associate Editor: Christine Tridente
Production Editor: Elizabeth Platt
Editorial Assistant: Thomas R. Prindle
Manufacturing Buyer: Amy Duddridge
Cover Design: Philip Regan
Design and Composition: D&G Limited, LLC
Printing and Binding: Courier Stoughton

Printed in the United States of America

10 09 08 07 06   10 9 8 7 6 5 4

THIS BOOK IS DEDICATED TO "MY BOYS"

ED,

BRIAN, SEAN, AND MICHAEL.

Contents

Appendixes

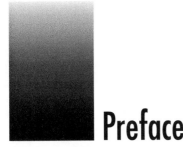

Preface

"Nursing faculty at our school have a part-time schedule. They only work twelve hours each day."
—Anonymous Nursing Faculty Member

There is a wealth of information available about educational assessment. Articles expressing concern about problems and posing approaches to various aspects of assessment and test development are replete in the current educational and nursing literature. In fact, many texts devote several chapters to issues related to assessment and classroom testing. However, until now there was no single, comprehensive resource devoted to the development of classroom exams as an integral aspect of a plan for the assessment of learning outcomes. This book is designed to do just that—to provide an all-inclusive reference that clarifies every aspect of the process for developing the most commonly used type of classroom assessment: the multiple-choice exam. Moreover, it focuses specifically on the development of valid and reliable multiple-choice exams in nursing education as a fundamental component of a plan for the systematic assessment of learning outcomes in the classroom setting.

The motivation for writing this book came from my experience as a nurse educator for more than 25 years. So many of the nursing students whom I have taught impressed me with their dedication to achieving competence in nursing. For many of those students, a nursing degree held a dual promise. It meant the fulfillment of a dream to enter a profession to which they were committed, and it also promised them, and their families, a secure future. However, many of these students were frustrated by their encounters with classroom testing and were confused by the way decisions were being made about the future that they were counting on so desperately.

At the same time, my colleagues and I were struggling to make student assessment decisions in a fair and honest manner. However, we did not always have as high a level of confidence in the decisions we were making as we would have preferred. Many times, this confusion and uneasiness led to conflict between students and faculty, and even among the faculty members.

An additional motive for writing this book stems from the requests made by numerous nursing programs for guidance in developing a plan for systematic educational assessment. Growing interest in educational assessment has emerged from the national concern for how well students are learning across all levels of education. In nursing, that concern is reflected in the accreditation standards established by national accreditation agencies. The accreditation standards of the National League for Nursing Accrediting Commission (NLNAC) require that nursing programs have an identified plan for systematic assessment of educational outcomes (NLNAC, 2000). One of the key elements of Standard IV (Program Effectiveness) of the accreditation standards from the Commission on Collegiate Nursing Education (CCNE) requires that faculty evaluation of student performance reflect the students' achievement of expected results (1998).

Purpose of the Book

In my experience, both as a nurse educator and as an educational assessment consultant, I have found that nursing faculty members are eager to improve their assessment skills. When I have held Test Development workshops at national nursing education conferences, there is usually "standing room only." In fact, at one meeting, the moveable walls actually had to be removed to allow for the overflow of nursing educators who demanded to be admitted to the session. This interest has made it clear to me that nursing faculty are aware of the implications of their student assessments, and they want to ensure that their methods are fair to the students whose lives are affected by their decisions.

Although teachers spend a great deal of time involved in assessment activities, teacher education in assessment theory is woefully inadequate at every level. As a result, many educators, including nurse educators, have taught themselves the skills for developing measurement instruments. This book attempts to fill the gap by providing nurse educators in both the education and practice settings with a resource for developing a valid and reliable assessment plan. Although it is not a comprehensive measurement text, you will find that this book includes extensive and detailed practical information about classroom test development. It is intended for the professional development of nurse educators, and it can also be a useful supplemental text in graduate programs for prospective nurse educators.

As a nurse educator you are faced with the challenge of making assessment decisions about students and you want to make those decisions objectively, with a high level of confidence. The key to attaining this high level of confidence is to establish a plan for systematic assessment so that you can base your decisions on valid and reliable measurement instruments. Most of you have prepared countless classroom tests and are well aware of the magnitude of that challenge and the responsibility that it entails. Yet, while you know what you want to assess, many of you are not confident in how to develop or interpret measurement instruments. This book will provide you with the necessary guidance to develop valid and reliable classroom multiple-choice exams as part of a systematic assessment plan, which will enable you to have the confidence level that is required for making important educational decisions about students.

The Prevalence of Multiple-Choice Exams

Because multiple-choice tests are so frequently used as the basis for classroom assessment, it is vital that nurse educators understand how to correctly develop them. Valid and reliable classroom test results are the product of a systematic plan that incorporates the principles of assessment. This book presents these principles, and it offers suggestions for producing that plan with a specific focus on the most widely used form of classroom assessment—the multiple-choice exam.

The principles reviewed in this book are the basic foundation of the development of a systematic assessment plan. Guidelines are offered to assist you in generating learning objectives and outcomes, developing blueprints, creating multiple-choice items, and analyzing overall test data as well as individual item responses. In following these suggestions, not only will you improve your classroom multiple-choice tests, you will also increase the quality of all of your student assessments.

For some, the material in the following chapters will be new; others will find that the book contains familiar information. Many of you may be tempted to skip ahead to Chapter 6, "Developing Multiple-Choice Items," eager to get started with the practical aspects of item development. However, I suggest that this is a mistake. You will never be able to develop effective multiple-choice items without first learning the preliminary steps of test development. While you cannot have a good test without good test items, it is also true that good test items evolve from a well-developed systematic assessment plan. In short, every educator who is involved in student assessment will benefit from reading the entire book. It contains an abundance of material that will enhance your understanding of the process of assessment, improve your multiple-choice item development skills, and ultimately benefit all of your assessment endeavors.

Critical Thinking Assessment

"Critical Thinking" is the contemporary educational buzz word. Teachers across the country at every educational level are concerned with how to promote and assess critical thinking across their curricula. One premise of this book is that there is a place for multiple-choice testing in assessing critical thinking.

The reality is that teacher-made multiple-choice exams are used extensively in education, particularly in nursing education. Despite its widespread use, the multiple-choice format has been criticized for failing to accurately measure higher-level cognitive abilities. While many testing experts agree that the multiple-choice format is the best tool for measuring knowledge, there is much debate about the role of this format for measuring complex cognitive ability, such as critical thinking (Haladyna, 1999). This book will demonstrate how multiple-choice tests can be developed to play a viable role in a multi-faceted approach for the assessment of higher-level thinking skills, including critical thinking in nursing.

Learning Curve

While nursing faculty are eager to improve their assessment skills, the difficulty that most of you express is how to fit yet another activity into your busy schedules. There is no doubt that nursing educators today are working on overload. After lecturing, clinical supervision, advisement, committee work, research, and publishing, it does seem that every minute of the day is accounted for. You might be concerned about how to squeeze yet another task into your busy schedule.

As with developing any new skill, or improving an old one, there is a learning curve associated with improving your assessment skills. However, I can assure you that the time you commit to developing an assessment system will benefit you many times over. At first, the forms and procedures may seem cumbersome. Yet, if you take the time to work with them for one semester, you will appreciate the benefit of a systematic approach to student assessment.

Chapter Synopsis

Chapter 1, "The Role of Assessment in Instruction," reviews the role of assessment in the educational process and the need for developing a plan for the systematic assessment of educational outcomes. The role of multiple-choice exams in that plan is identified and the ethical responsibilities associated with classroom testing and the implications of assessment decisions on the lives of students are discussed. Assessment competency standards are reviewed and the need for improving teacher skills in the development of multiple-choice classroom exams is also addressed.

Assessment terminology is reviewed in Chapter 2, "The Language of Assessment." An overview of the principles of assessment is presented, and the common language associated with educational assessment is reviewed and explained. (Many of these concepts are elaborated on in subsequent chapters.) The discussion in this chapter focuses on the essential nature of reliability and validity in the process of test development, and it enumerates the factors that impact these properties.

The role of objectives as the foundation for the instructional process is presented in Chapter 3, "Developing Instructional Objectives." Guidelines for developing objectives and learning outcomes and criteria for writing effective objectives are proposed. The chapter also identifies the characteristics of mastery- and developmental-level objectives and addresses the application of strategies to assess those objectives.

Critical thinking in nursing is discussed in Chapter 4, "Assessing Critical Thinking." The need for developing a definition of the construct is discussed and the characteristics of critical thinking, as identified in the nursing literature, are reviewed. A definition of critical thinking is proposed as a basis for objective test development, and an instructional objective is developed from that definition. The challenge of assessing critical thinking is also addressed along with the identification of specific critical thinking behaviors that can be translated into multiple-choice items.

Chapter 5, "Implementing Systematic Test Development," examines the process of developing a multiple-choice test and proposes a systematic approach for outlining content and blueprint development. In addition, the NCLEX-RN test plan is reviewed and several cross-reference tables are provided. This chapter also addresses the issue of student preparation for a test.

Chapter 6, "Developing Multiple-Choice Items," continues the discussion of test development by analyzing the advantages and disadvantages of multiple-choice exams. The characteristics of effective multiple-choice items are examined in detail and guidelines are also proposed for improving item writing. Numerous item examples are offered and strategies for framing questions and conducting peer review are suggested.

Chapter 7, "Writing Critical Thinking Multiple-Choice Items," builds on the previous chapters to present the issues associated with the creation of critical thinking multiple-choice items. The characteristics of critical thinking multiple-choice items are presented, and specific examples directly related to previously established learning outcomes are offered. Strategies for crafting multiple-choice items, which assess critical thinking, are proposed.

Issues related to assembling, administering, and scoring a test are addressed in Chapter 8, "Assembling, Administering, and Scoring a Test." Concerns such as cheating and maintaining test security throughout the testing process are discussed. The chapter also deals with the considerations for qualitative peer review, student post-test review, and student challenges to exam questions.

Chapter 9, "Establishing Evidence of Reliability and Validity," examines the issue of documenting the reliability and validity of a test. Measures of reliability and the effects of measurement error are discussed. Validity is also examined as a crucial ingredient for teacher confidence in assessment decisions. Statistical formulas are presented for those who appreciate a mathematical explanation of the concepts of reliability and validity.

A careful test analysis is a prerequisite for assigning objective scores to a multiple-choice exam. Both qualitative and quantitative analyses contribute to fair evaluation of a measurement instrument. Chapter 10, "Interpreting Test Results," explains the meaning of the statistics included in a test data report as the basis for translating raw test scores into fair grade assignments. Individual item analysis is also carefully examined both as a test analysis tool and for its value in guiding the improvement of existing items.

One of the most difficult aspects of the teacher's role is grading. Chapter 11, "Assigning Grades" examines how a grading plan evolves from the principles of grading and a teacher's personal grading philosophy. Practical suggestions for implementing a grading plan, including issues such as using an absolute versus a relative standard, are explored.

Chapter 12, "Instituting Item Banking and Test Development Software," concludes the book with practical suggestions and examples for improving items based on item analysis, establishing an item bank, and for implementing test development software. The chapter presents a comprehensive overview of the requirements for utilizing a system to streamline the development and improvement of multiple-choice items. The objective of this chapter is to consolidate the important information that will help you expedite the process of implementing these programs.

This book translates the principles and practices of assessment into guidelines that will assist you in developing a plan for the systematic assessment of learning outcomes. Although the focus of the book is on developing multiple-choice exams as the basis for that plan, following these guidelines will improve your overall assessment plan. While I strongly suggest that you read the book from cover to cover, it is also intended to be a working reference. It is not meant to be read once and put on your bookshelf. There is considerable overlap in the components of the assessment process. Therefore, some aspects are addressed in more than one chapter. This repetition is meant to keep the process clear and to provide you with a reference that is easy to access when you are in the process of developing a test.

Developing a systematic plan for the assessment of learning outcomes is a challenge. Creating effective multiple-choice exams, which supports that plan, is a skill that develops with a concentrated effort over time. As with all aspects of the educational process, there are no hard and fast assessment "rules." However, you should seriously consider adopting the guidelines suggested in the following chapters because they are based on generally agreed upon opinions of measurement experts.

The instruments of assessment are open to interpretation. Ultimately, it is your professional judgment that will bring all of the pieces together to form your assessment plan. This book is designed to assist you in developing measurement instruments, particularly multiple-choice exams, on which you can confidently base your assessment decisions.

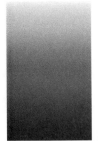

Acknowledgments

Writing a book is a unique experience; a challenge that cannot be appreciated until it is attempted. This particular attempt would never have been accomplished had it not been for the advice and support of my colleagues, friends, and family.

I am especially grateful for the suggestions of my colleagues who generously offered their time to review the manuscript with care and attention to detail. A special thanks goes to Joanne Lavin who, in the midst of her own busy schedule, read every draft of every chapter. Her insightful comments and encouragement motivated me to continue this endeavor. Arthur Ellen provided invaluable advice, which helped me to refine the chapters related to reliability and validity. Margaret Rafferty shared her test development and item banking expertise for every chapter, and Maureen Esteves and Donna Knauth offered their suggestions from the viewpoint of nursing faculty. Veronica Phillips-Arikian painstakingly read the entire manuscript and shared her testing expertise to improve the final draft. Finally, I would like to thank my son, Sean, who helped clarify the complicated statistical explanations.

Thanks to my sons, my students, and my colleagues who have been the inspiration for this book. Most of all, thanks to my husband, Ed, whose support and encouragement has afforded me the luxury of pursuing my passion.

1 The Role of Assessment in Instruction

> *"We're having a test in school tomorrow, and there's no way*
> *I can pass it . . . Absolutely no way!"*
>
> —Charlie Brown
> Peanuts (1968)

The ability to think critically in order to provide therapeutic nursing care is one of the most important outcomes of nursing education. While nurse educators are proficient at developing creative instructional strategies to assist students in attaining this outcome, they frequently are not as adept at creating instruments that effectively measure it. As a result, assessment of critical thinking frequently receives inadequate attention within the instructional process.

Although assessment is an integral component of the instructional process, teachers often pay more attention to the content of a course than to the process of assessment. For many educators, preparing assessments is an arduous task. Some even feel that evaluation is the antithesis of teaching; that the role of evaluator is at odds with the role of educator; that tests are a necessary evil; and that assessments are less important than instruction. These perceptions could not be any further from reality. Teaching is not automatically effective. Assessment provides valuable information about student achievement and also assists educators in determining the effectiveness of their instructional strategies.

The Nature of Assessment

Assessment is the systematic process of collecting and interpreting information to make an informed decision. Popham defines educational assessment as "a formal attempt to determine students' status with respect to educational variables of interest"

(1999, p. 3). All assessments begin with a purpose. Classroom assessment is a formal process that involves a deliberate effort to gain information about a student's status in relation to educational variables such as knowledge, attitudes, and skills. This process includes a wide range of procedures, and has the ultimate goal of obtaining valid and reliable information on which educational decisions can be based.

Planning, teaching, and assessment are viewed as the three interactive components of educational instruction (Brookhart, 1999). Planning involves the establishment of behavioral objectives and learning outcomes, which leads to decisions about the types of instructional activities that will enable students to successfully achieve the required outcomes. The desired learning outcomes and instructional activities then guide the assessment techniques, while the assessment results should direct and even modify the teaching approach. Figure 1.1 illustrates this relationship, which Brookhart (1999) describes as effective when the assessment instruments are valid, reliable, and provide accurate, meaningful, and appropriate information.

PLANNING

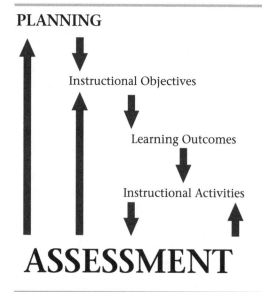

ASSESSMENT

FIGURE 1.1   Interaction of planning, teaching, and assessment in educational instruction.

While the main goal of classroom assessment is to obtain valid, reliable, and useful information about student achievement, assessment procedures also assist in appraising the effectiveness of the instruction. A well-designed assessment plan will help you to identify your own strengths and weaknesses and will guide your teaching approach. The results of a classroom test based on such a plan can also provide answers to the following questions:

- What is the level of the students' achievement?

- Are the course objectives realistic?

- Are the instruction methods appropriate?

- How well are the learning experiences sequenced?

In addition to being the primary indicator of student achievement and the effectiveness of an educational program, student assessment is also an integral part of the learning process. Effective assessment is a continuous process, which provides valuable feedback for students, thus reinforcing successful learning and offering information about further learning needs. While poorly designed assessment is at odds with learning, assessment that is well designed not only promotes learning, but also enhances teaching by assisting both the student in learning and the teacher in teaching (Mehrens & Lehmann, 1973). Well-developed classroom assessments contribute to effective student learning by helping students identify their strengths and weaknesses to guide their future study.

All too often, students feel that no matter what they do, they will not be able to pass classroom exams. Unfortunately, these perceptions of teacher-made tests are frequently correct. Poorly constructed, teacher-made tests frustrate students and can undermine their self-confidence. No doubt you have heard a student say, "There is no way that I can pass this test." When tests are perceived as unfair or too difficult, many students will protect their self-esteem by giving up, rather than repeatedly fail. When students do fail, educators must first ask themselves if the instructional process contributed to the failure.

Ethical Responsibility

Educators have an ethical responsibility every time they assess students. Basic to this responsibility is the recognition that assessment is a means to an end, not an end in itself. It is essential that students realize that educators do not assess people, they assess characteristics of people. Assessment should never be confused with measuring the worth of an individual (Meherns & Lehmann, 1973), by either teachers or students.

Teacher-made tests play a central role in student assessment. In light of the influence that decisions based on these tests have on the lives of students, elaborate care must be taken when testing and grading. Decisions about promotion, placement, retention, and graduation are often based on teacher-made classroom assessments. These decisions have such meaningful consequences for students that teachers are ethically bound to provide defensible evidence of the reliability and validity of their classroom assessments (Airasian, 1997). Educators should work equally as hard at developing fair assessments and assigning fair and accurate grades as the students work to obtain them.

Fundamental to the development of valid assessments is the recognition that test preparation in the classroom deserves the same priority as the preparation of classroom instruction. Consider the amount of group effort that is invested in the development of a course in a nursing program. Endless meetings and discussions are held to write objectives and content outlines and to plan learning activities. Yet, test development is often a solitary process, with individual faculty members contributing pieces to the final product, without even seeing the whole picture.

As Clements and MacDonald (1966) explain, ethical responsibility for student assessment requires teachers to assure that each assessment tool

- Is appropriately designed

- Actually measures what it claims to measure

In addition, Clements and MacDonald also point out that when interpreting the results of assessment instruments, teachers must seriously consider the following:

- Emotional and social impact on students
- Consequences of the evaluation on a student's academic life

Assessment and Self-Efficacy

One of the most important responsibilities of a teacher is to help students to maximize their success and to promote every student's self-efficacy. In order to promote self-efficacy, which can be described as the *I can do it* attitude, teachers need to believe that every student can be successful (Haladyna, 1999). Admission to a nursing program is certainly a selective process and every admitted student has the potential for success. It is the obligation of the program's faculty to assist every student in becoming successful.

In the process of promoting student self-efficacy, it is important to remember that a student's sense of accomplishment will be diminished if a task is too easy and will be defeated if a task is too hard (Haladyna, 1999). When tests are perceived as trivial, students perceive school work as trivial and can adopt the attitude that the process of learning is one of passive recall. We cannot expect students to be successful, to have the *I can do it* attitude on *high stakes* exams, such as the National Council Licensure Exam (NCLEX), if they are accustomed to taking poorly constructed classroom exams that are perceived as too easy or too difficult.

It is unrealistic to think that a post-program review course can teach students to be successful on a national exam. The best approach for fostering a realistic sense of self-efficacy is to expose students throughout their entire nursing program to well-constructed tests that require them to think critically and to apply their acquired knowledge.

How many multiple-choice exams do students take over the course of a nursing program—20, 30, 50? It is certainly not unusual for students to answer more than 2,000 multiple-choice items during a nursing program. By presenting them with well-written exams that assess higher-order thinking, nursing programs can challenge students' critical thinking ability and provide them with the best preparation for passing the NCLEX licensure exam.

Assessment Inadequacy

Although most teachers recognize and strive to fulfill their assessment role, many experience conflict originating from feelings of inadequacy. These feelings of assessment inadequacy are understandable. While assessment is integral to instruction and learning, classroom assessment and grading are generally acknowledged as the weak links in modern education. Despite the widespread use of classroom achievement tests and the important role they play in the instructional process, teachers of all disciplines at every level lack the understanding of assessment methods. Surveys of teacher preparation (Impara, 1995; Stiggins, 1999) have reported that teachers are often ill-prepared in the development and use of classroom assessments. Despite the fact that classroom assessment is an integral part of a teacher's responsibility, many have not received the basic instruction in the process of assessment and grading that is necessary for fair student evaluation (Haladyna, 1997).

Nursing education is facing a particular dilemma with the assessment competency of faculty. Even in 1980, Fitzpatrick and Heller identified that the number of nurses with the necessary preparation in education was dwindling. That trend has continued over the last twenty years. Expert clinicians, rather than educators, have increasingly been filling nurse faculty positions. Although these faculty members have valuable clinical expertise, they lack the preparation for the role of teacher, which includes assessment proficiency (Choudhry, 1992; Davis, Dearman, Schwab, & Kitchens, 1992; DeYoung & Beshore-Bliss, 1995).

The current national trend of increasing the number of graduate programs designed for expanded clinical nursing roles will only exacerbate the problem of an increasing population of nursing faculty who are not adequately prepared for their educational roles. An obvious long-term solution is to incorporate educational preparation into all graduate nurse education. However, in the meantime, workshops and continuing education programs are necessary to upgrade the assessment competency of nursing faculty.

Assessment Competency Standards

As public and professional awareness of the need for assessment competence increases, several professional organizations have developed standards to provide guidelines for the assessment skills that educators should possess. The most recent edition of *The Standards for Educational and Psychological Testing* was jointly developed by the American Educational Research Association (AERA), the American Psychological Association (APA), and the National Council on Measurement in Education (NCME). The intent of this document is to "promote the sound and ethical use of tests and to provide a basis for evaluating the quality of testing practices" (1999, p. 1). These standards represent a consensus on the skills required of teachers that enable them to appropriately use educational and psychological tests. An ad hoc committee of the NCME published the *Code of Professional Responsibilities in Educational Measurement* in 1995 in order to "promote professionally responsible practice in educational measurement" (p. 2). Both of these documents provide valuable guidelines for fair and ethical assessment in higher education.

The *Standards for Teacher Competence in Educational Assessment of Students* (1990) was jointly developed by the American Federation of Teachers (AFT), the National Council on Measurement in Education (NCME), and the National Education Association (NEA). This collaboration between teaching and measurement specialists defined seven assessment competencies (summarized in Table 1.1) that are critical to the role of educator. While these standards were specifically written for K–12 classroom teachers, they also provide a discussion model for professional competence and fairness in assessment in higher education (Brookhart, 1999).

Unfortunately, the assessment abilities of many teachers are often inconsistent with the standards that have been adopted by professional organizations (Impara, 1995). The assessment content presented in this book is consistent with those professional standards and will provide you with a foundation for achieving competence in student assessment.

TABLE 1.1   Standards for Teacher Competence in Educational Assessment

Teachers should be skilled in

1. Choosing assessment methods appropriate for instructional decisions.

2. Developing assessment methods appropriate for instructional decisions.

3. Administering, scoring, and interpreting the results of both externally-produced and teacher-produced assessment methods.

4. Using assessment results when making decisions about individual students, planning teaching, developing curriculum, and school improvement.

5. Developing valid pupil grading procedures which use pupil assessments.

6. Communicating assessment results to students, parents, other lay audiences, and other educators.

7. Recognizing unethical, illegal, and otherwise inappropriate assessment methods and uses of assessment information.

Source: American Federation of Teachers, National Council on Measurement in Education, National Education Association (1990). *Standard for Teacher Competence in Educational Assessment of Students.* Washington, D.C.: National Council on Measurement in Education.

The Need for a Systematic Approach to Assessment

A systematic plan is defined as a procedure that is based on a coordinated method. It ensures that no steps are omitted from a process. The only way to ensure that all steps are completed in a complicated process is by following a system. The nursing process provides an example of a systematic method applied to a complex process. Certainly, there is no process more complex than the practice of nursing. Widely adopted by the profession, particularly in nursing education, the nursing process provides a systematic approach that ensures the comprehensive application of nursing care.

As you will see, a comprehensive assessment plan involves several interacting processes. In order to maintain the plan's integrity, a methodical procedure, which is based on the principles of assessment, must be designed and followed. In fact, having a defined methodology will not only ensure that steps are not missing, but will also ensure that objectivity is maintained throughout the assessment process.

In fact, following a systematic procedure for each of the components of the overall plan will assure that your assessment plan is both comprehensive and objective. This book is designed to help you develop a system that will streamline every aspect of your assessment plan. Not only will the guidelines ensure that your plan is practical and comprehensive, but they will also ensure that it is grounded in the principles of sound assessment.

Assessment Instruments

As defined in Standard One of the *Standards for Teacher Competence in Educational Assessment of Students* (1990), when planning assessment strategies, it is important that you choose the assessment technique appropriate for the particular behavior being assessed. Brookhart (1999) describes the following four categories of assessment instruments:

- Paper-and-pencil tests
- Performance assessments
- Oral communications
- Portfolio assessment

A multidimensional approach is essential in order to assess all aspects of a behavior. This is especially true when assessing psychomotor skills, affective behavior, or higher-level cognitive ability, such as critical thinking. For a variety of reasons, multiple-choice paper-and-pencil classroom tests, which are developed by teachers, are widely used in all educational settings, particularly in nursing education. The focus of this book is on the role of the multiple-choice format for classroom tests as part of a multidimensional plan for assessment of learning outcomes. This book provides you with the strategies you need to develop well-constructed, valid, and reliable multiple-choice exams.

Summary

Assessment is integral to the instructional process. While nursing faculty have the ethical responsibility to ensure that student assessments are properly designed and administered, the assessment part of the instructional process often does not receive the attention it deserves. There are several reasons for the neglect of assessment. One of the most important reasons is the need for faculty to have increased awareness of assessment principles and techniques.

This book provides nursing educators with a review of the theories and principles of assessment. Practical guidelines for developing valid and reliable multiple-choice classroom tests are offered. The intent is not to present the multiple-choice format as superior, or even equal, to other formats for all types of assessment. However, because multiple-choice exams are so prevalent in nursing education, it is essential that faculty become familiar with the strategies they need to create valid and reliable tests.

This book is designed to help you to develop a systematic plan for assessment of learning outcomes. It demonstrates how valid and reliable multiple-choice exams are one method for assessing critical thinking in nursing. Assessment issues are addressed and practical guidelines are presented to assist you in developing multiple-choice exams that reflect the standards of assessment competence. In addition to improving your multiple-choice exams, the information presented in the following chapters will also assist you in improving your overall assessment program, no matter which assessment format you choose to implement.

2 The Language of Assessment

"To teach without testing is unthinkable."
—American Association of School Administrators

Assessment, measurement, evaluation, test. These are terms that are often used interchangeably. Although they are closely linked in the process of developing an assessment plan, each has a distinct role. Familiarity with the terminology of assessment will facilitate your understanding of the bigger picture. The purpose of this chapter is to review the basic principles of assessment. It will provide you with a clear understanding of the framework on which a comprehensive systematic assessment plan is based, and how valid and reliable multiple-choice exams are developed. Many of these concepts will be addressed in detail in subsequent chapters.

Most of you will be familiar with these terms. Some readers may even prefer to move past this chapter and delve right into the strategies for developing multiple-choice items. However, as the book demonstrates, you cannot start writing multiple-choice items until your assessment plan is established. Unless you consistently work in the area of assessment, you will find this refresher beneficial. Reviewing this chapter will increase your fluency in the Language of Assessment, and your understanding of the proposed guidelines.

Assessment

Chapter 1, "The Role of Assessment in Instruction," introduces you to the concept of assessment as a broad and comprehensive process of collecting quantitative and qualitative data to make informed educational decisions. It is a process that encompasses the full range of procedures used to obtain information about student learning. Data collection for assessment should be directed by clearly defined learning targets or objectives (Nitko, 1996). In nursing education, assessment answers the question: "How well has the student achieved the learning objectives?"

Nitko (1996) proposes a set of five principles to help guide teachers in the selection and use of classroom assessments. Nitko's principles (pp.4-6) provide a basis for developing a plan for systematic assessment of learning outcomes:

1. IDENTIFY the desired learning targets (outcomes). In order to select the appropriate assessment techniques, the behaviors that represent achievement of the objectives must be clearly defined.

2. ASSURE that the selected assessment techniques match the learning outcomes. While assessment techniques should be practical and efficient, it is more important that they are derived from the intellectual challenge posed by the learning outcomes.

3. PROVIDE assessment opportunities that meet a learner's needs. Students should be given concrete examples of what is expected of them and the assessment techniques should provide meaningful feedback.

4. EMPLOY multiple measurement techniques to assess each learning outcome. The validity of assessment is enhanced by using multiple assessment modalities. A variety of measurements may be required to evaluate whether a student has attained a particular learning outcome, especially if the outcome involves higher-order thinking.

5. CONSIDER the limitations of assessment techniques when interpreting their results. It is important to remember that the information obtained, even when multiple assessment techniques are used, is only a sample of a student's behavior, and that the interpretation of all assessments is subject to measurement error.

Measurement

Measurement is defined as the process of determining the extent to which some trait, characteristic, or behavior is associated with a person (McMillan, 1997). It encompasses a variety of techniques, including tests, ratings, and observations, which are designed to assign a score that represents the degree of a pre-defined trait that an individual possesses. Thus, measurements provide the information to guide decision making. While valid measurements contribute to valid decisions, erroneous measures can lead to inappropriate decisions. Therefore, it is imperative for educators to ensure that their measurement instruments are sound.

Objectivity is an essential element of a reliable and valid measurement. If a measurement is not objective, the measurement's results depend more on the subjective opinion of the person who is conducting the measurement rather than on the ability of the person who is being measured. In order for a measurement instrument to be objective, it must be confined to assigning a number or a rating to a student characteristic based on pre-defined, objective evidence of the characteristic.

One common measurement error is to equate quantification with objective measurement. Numbers have a scientific quality that can be confused with objectivity. Just because a measurement instrument produces a numerical score does not mean that the score is an objective one. A score of 80 on a test is meaningless and arbitrary if the score is based on a test that was poorly constructed in the first place.

Assessment instruments that provide qualitative information are sometimes chosen as the most desirable instruments for classroom measurement. When an assessment involves a procedure that describes student achievement in qualitative terms, extreme care must be taken to assure objectivity when assigning a number or category as a score. Whatever technique you choose, it is essential that your measurements are never based on subjective judgments.

In addition, it is very important to acknowledge that measurement skills are not intuitive. The ability to produce valid and reliable measurements is acquired and develops with practice. One way to immediately improve your measurement skills is to follow the four steps for developing effective classroom measurement instruments (as shown in Table 2.1). The following chapters will examine each of these steps in detail.

TABLE 2.1   Steps for Developing Effective Measurement Instruments

1. Identify the instructional objectives and learning outcomes.

2. Develop a blueprint based on those outcomes.

3. Create items to measure the outcomes.

4. Quantify the results of the measurement.

Note that Step 1 in Table 2.1 reflects the first of Nitko's (1996) assessment guidelines: Identify the desired learning targets. This is also the first step in the development of a systematic plan for assessment. As you read this book, you will recognize that the steps for developing an assessment plan overlap, and that each reflects Nitko's assessment guidelines.

Evaluation

Measurement and evaluation are not equivalent. Evaluation is defined as a judgment that appraises and attaches meaning to the data obtained through measurement. It is guided by professional judgment and involves comparing a measurement to a standard and making a decision based on that comparison. The standard or outcomes that students are expected to achieve must be established at the beginning of the instructional process. Establishing the behavior standards and clearly communicating them to the students facilitates the evaluation of students' achievement of the learning outcomes. Table 2.2 exemplifies the difference between measurement and evaluation.

TABLE 2.2   The Difference between Measurement and Evaluation

Measurement: The student correctly answered 85 out of 100 items on the multiple-choice exam.

Evaluation: The student performed at an above average level.

While evaluation involves a judgment about the merit of an individual's performance, it also involves a judgment about the value of the measurement. Although fair evaluation should be objective, classroom evaluation tends to be subjective because human judgment is subjective. Therefore, it is a teacher's responsibility to verify that evaluation is based on objective assessments. The more judgments are based on carefully constructed and administered classroom measurement instruments, the greater the likelihood that they will be objectively sound. Furthermore, the more familiarity you have with the principles of assessment, the greater your confidence will be in the objectivity and ultimate fairness of your evaluations.

Formative Evaluation

Formative evaluation directs future learning by appraising the quality of student achievement while the student is still in the process of learning. It judges student progress toward meeting instructional objectives with the intent of improving teaching and learning. Formative evaluation is diagnostic evaluation—it identifies students' strengths and weaknesses to provide feedback for improvement of teaching and learning. Because formative evaluation is a method that shapes the process of teaching and learning while it is in progress, it is usually not used for assigning class grades.

Summative Evaluation

The focus of summative evaluation is to describe the quality of student achievement after an instructional process is completed. While a formative evaluation asks, "How are you doing?", summative evaluation asks, "How did you do?" (Slavin, 1997, p. 491). A summative evaluation is given at the conclusion of a unit or a course of instruction, and it focuses on determining whether learning has occurred and if the desired outcomes have been achieved. Summative evaluation provides a summary of student achievement and is used to determine students' grades and their progress in an educational program.

Summative and formative evaluation should be consistent. This consistency is achieved when both are based on the instructional objectives established at the beginning of the course. In addition, it is imperative that students know if an evaluation is formative or summative so they will understand if this evaluation is for practice, or if grades will be assigned. Table 2.3 compares formative and summative evaluation.

Instructional Objectives

The first step in the development of an assessment plan is the careful preparation of the instructional objectives and learning outcomes. Clearly defined objectives identify the student behavior, which is going to be assessed, and specify what a student should know and be able to do at the end of an instructional course (Gronlund, 2000). As Robert Mager stated, "When clearly defined goals are lacking, it is impossible to evaluate a course or program efficiently, and there is no sound basis for selecting appropriate materials, content, or instructional methods" (1962, p. 3). The development of instructional objectives and learning outcomes is the focus of Chapter 3, "Developing Instructional Objectives."

TABLE 2.3   Comparison of Formative and Summative Evaluation

Formative Evaluation	Summative Evaluation
How are you doing?	**How did you do?**
• Occurs during the process of learning	• Occurs at the completion of instruction
• Assesses progress in a course	• Summarizes achievement in a course
• Directs learning to achieve objectives	• Assesses objective achievement
• Grades not assigned	• Assigns grades
• Provides feedback	• Provides feedback

Learning Outcomes

The most effective way to state instructional objectives is in terms of the behaviors that you expect students to achieve by the end of a course. Gronlund (2000) maintains that defining objectives in terms of desired student learning outcomes shifts the focus from the learning process to the learning outcomes, and also provides a basis for the assessment of student learning. Gronlund also suggests that stating the general objective first and then listing a representational sample of learning outcomes clarifies to the student what has been deemed acceptable by the teacher as evidence that the student has attained the objective.

Blueprint

A blueprint, also referred to as a table of specifications or test plan, is the foundation for establishing content-related evidence of validity for a test. A test cannot include the entire instructional domain of a course, yet it should include a representative sample of that specific domain. A blueprint is defined as a mechanism that guides the systematic selection of a representative sample of the content and objectives of a course. A test based on a carefully planned blueprint will enable you to project that a student who receives a score of 90 percent on a 50-item test would receive a score of 90 percent on a 500-item test.

Content validation of a classroom achievement test involves collecting evidence to evaluate the degree to which the test reflects the course's instructional objectives and content. Establishing content-related evidence of validity must begin with test development. It only makes sense to plan ahead. To make sure that a test represents the desired outcomes of a course, it must be based on a blueprint. The blueprint guides the selection of test questions that reflect achievement of the content and course objectives.

A blueprint answers the question, "What is being measured?" Although a blueprint directs the selection of test items, it is still the teacher's responsibility to carefully plan and develop these items so that they actually measure student ability in the areas specified by the blueprint. Blueprints can be developed for a variety of measurement techniques—to enable the selection of the most appropriate instrument to measure the attainment of the course objectives, content, and skills.

Test development is a time-consuming process. However, using a blueprint as a guide expedites this process and provides the structure for creating valid and reliable tests. The effort required for plan development is time well spent. In the long run, it will facilitate test development and increase your confidence in the decisions you make based on your measurement instruments. Chapter 5, "Implementing Systematic Test Development," provides you with detailed guidelines for blueprint development.

Item Bank

An item bank is defined as an organized collection of items that can be accessed for test development. Testing experts often distinguish between item *pools* and item *banks*. This distinction defines a bank as a set of items whose difficulty levels have been calibrated on a common scale; while a pool simply consists of a collection of items. Because the term *item bank* is commonly used in test development software designed for classroom use, it is used throughout this book. Although a classroom item bank is designed to accumulate item data, the difficulty levels of the items in the classroom item banks referred to in the following chapters are not calibrated. The implementation of an item banking program is closely examined in Chapter 12, "Instituting Item Banking and Test Development Software."

Test

Tests are measurement instruments; formal events where individuals are asked to demonstrate their achievement of some knowledge or skill in a specific domain. The purpose of an achievement test is to obtain relevant and accurate data needed to make important decisions with a minimum amount of error. It is assumed that students have achieved learning objectives when a designated test score is obtained. Tests that are well designed and appropriately used can contribute to more effective teaching and learning (Gronlund, 1993).

Using a single test or type of measurement instrument is not a satisfactory assessment strategy. Most course objectives require a variety of measurement and evaluation strategies to determine student competency in a particular course. The selection of measurement instruments depends on the outcomes to be measured. It is important to select the most appropriate strategies for measuring each learning outcome. One premise of this book is that multiple-choice exams can be developed to contribute to the assessment of objectives that require higher-level cognitive ability, including the construct of critical thinking.

An achievement test should consist of a sampling of tasks, which represents the larger domain of behavior that is being assessed (Gronlund, 1993). When students complain that an exam did not cover the course content, it may indicate that there is a mismatch between the test items and the larger domain of course content or objectives; or it may indicate that the items did not address the designated content or objectives. It is not possible to measure a student's achievement of objectives with items that do not match those particular objectives. Therefore, the challenge is to develop a blueprint for the test and write items to match the objectives and content being assessed.

Interpreting Test Scores

A raw test score is meaningless without a framework for interpretation. The raw test score is only given meaning within the instructional content domain it represents. Criterion-referenced tests assess an individual's performance based on the percentage of the content mastered. Norm-referenced tests define an individual's performance by comparing it to others. Although both types of interpretation can be applied to the same test, the interpretation is most meaningful when the test is specifically designed for a desired interpretation (Linn & Gronlund, 2000).

Criterion-Referenced Tests

Criterion-referenced tests (CRTs) interpret a student's raw score using a preset standard established by the faculty. Thus, each student's competency in relation to the preset standard is measured without reference to any other student. Student scores are then reported as the percentage correct with each student's performance level determined by the preset, or absolute, standard. Figure 2.1 presents an example of a criterion-referenced objective.

The student demonstrated mastery by correctly identifying 90 percent of the terms.

FIGURE 2.1   Example of a criterion-referenced score

Because CRTs measure a student's attainment of a set of learning outcomes, no attempt should be made to eliminate easy items. The content chosen for a CRT depends only on how well it matches the learning outcomes of the course (Bond, 1996). If most of the students in a group meet the standard, the group scores will obviously cluster at the high end of the grading scale.

CRTs are often teacher-made and are closely tied to the objectives and curriculum. They are most meaningful when they are specifically designed to measure student ability in a particular area (Gronlund, 1973). Competency is such a critical requirement in nursing education that CRT is often the preferred form of classroom testing in nursing education (Reilly & Oermann, 1990).

Gronlund describes the relationship of criterion-referenced testing to the two levels of learning: mastery and developmental (1973). Designing tests for these two different levels of learning poses different challenges.

MASTERY LEVEL LEARNING   At this level, criterion-referenced tests are concerned with measuring the minimum essential skills that indicate mastery of an objective. The scope of learning tasks is limited, which simplifies the process of assessment. A score of the percentage correct is usually used to identify how closely a student's score demonstrates a complete mastery of an objective. One challenge for the faculty is to identify 1) which specific learning outcomes the students are expected to master, and 2) which objectives represent learning beyond the mastery level, or developmental learning (Gronlund, 1973). Chapters 3, "Developing Instructional Objectives," and 4, "Assessing Critical Thinking," offer a more in-depth discussion and also provide examples of objectives at the mastery and developmental levels of learning.

DEVELOPMENTAL LEVEL LEARNING   The concept of developmental learning applies to constructs that represent complex, higher-order thinking, such as critical thinking. The abilities associated with this level are continuously developing throughout life. Developmental level objectives represent goals to work toward, with emphasis focused on continuous development, rather than a complete mastery of a set of predetermined skills (Gronlund, 1973).

Learning outcomes at the developmental level represent degrees of progress toward an objective. Because it is impossible to identify all of the behaviors that represent a complex construct, only a sample of the behaviors associated with instructional objectives at this level can be identified as learning outcomes. These behaviors should define the construct and provide a representational sample of student performance that will be accepted as evidence of the appropriate progress toward the attainment of the ultimate objective.

Students are not expected to fully achieve objectives at the developmental level. However, they are required to demonstrate the behaviors represented by the learning outcomes, and they are also encouraged to strive for their personal level of maximum achievement toward the ultimate objective—their *personal best*. At this level, instructional objectives can be designed to show the development of students as they progress through an instructional program. For example, the same general instructional objectives can be used in every course in a nursing program, with the learning outcomes becoming more complex as the students progress through the program.

Gronlund asserts that the use of criterion-referenced tests is restricted with the assessment of developmental learning. While test preparation should follow mastery-level procedures, he suggests that in order to adequately describe student performance beyond minimal essentials, tests at the developmental level should include items of varying difficulty and allow for both criterion and norm-referenced interpretations (1973).

Norm-Referenced Tests

While CRTs measure a student's achievement of a program's objectives without reference to other students, the aim of norm-referenced tests (NRTs) is to compare a student's achievement to the achievement of the student's peer group. NRTs focus on a student's performance in relation to other students, rather than in relation to the attainment of a course's objectives. Norms themselves do not represent levels of performance—they provide a frame of reference to use when comparing the performances of a group of individuals. NRTs interpret a student's raw score as a percentile rank in a group. NRTs do not indicate what a student has achieved, the tests only indicate how the student compares to other students in their group. An example of a norm-referenced score is shown in Figure 2.2.

The student's performance equaled or exceeded 82 percent of the students in the group.

FIGURE 2.2   Example of a norm-referenced score

NRTs are designed to discriminate between strong and weak students. The tests are designed to provide a wide range of scores so that the identification of students at different achievement levels is possible. Therefore, items that all students are likely to answer correctly are eliminated.

The content selected for an NRT is based on how well it ranks students from high to low achievers (Bond, 1996). The NRT format is commonly used on national standardized tests. These tests have a generalized content that is commonly taught in many schools. The norms established by a standardized achievement test are based on nationally accepted educational goals, which enable educators to compare a student's test score to the scores of other students in similar programs in the United States. These scores provide a general indication of the strengths and weaknesses of the students in a particular school, and afford faculty an external reference point for comparing their curriculum to a composite national curriculum.

NRTs in the classroom setting identify how students compare to each other. Because strict NRTs are not concerned with the level of individual student achievement, they are usually not appropriate for classroom use. When assessing developmental learning, Gronlund suggests using NRTs to rank students with the addition of criterion-referenced interpretations applied to the test to assess degrees of student progress toward an objective (1973). Table 2.4 compares CRTs and NRTs.

TABLE 2.4   Comparison of Criterion- and Norm-Referenced Tests

Criterion-Referenced Test	Norm-Referenced Test
• Compares student performance to pre-established criteria	• Compares student performance to reference group
• Describes the performance	• Discriminates the performance
• Mastery reference	• Relative performance reference
• Narrowly-defined content domain	• More diverse content domain
• Larger number of items for each objective	• Smaller number of items for each objective
• Includes easy items	• Eliminates easy items
• Focuses on student competency	• Focuses on student ranking
• Provides percent-correct score	• Provides percentile rank

Grade

While a test score is a numerical indication of what is observed from a single measurement instrument, a grade is a label representing a composite evaluation. A course grade should be derived from the accumulation of scores obtained from several measurement instruments. Because life-altering decisions are associated with student grades, the utmost care must be used when assigning test scores and grades. Chapters 10, "Interpreting Test Results," and 11, "Assigning Grades," discuss test analysis and grading procedures.

Test Bias

A biased test is one that discriminates against a certain group based on socioeconomic status, disability, race, ethnicity, or gender (Slavin, 1997). Test bias refers to the difference in a group's mean performance based on an unfair measurement. When a measurement is biased, students who have the same ability perform differently on the same task because of their affiliation with a particular ethnic, sexual, cultural, or religious group. (Hambleton & Rodgers, 1996). Hambleton and Rodgers define stereotyping as another undesirable characteristic of a test that introduces bias. Stereotyping refers to the representation of a group in such a manner that it may be offensive to the group members. They also note that test language that is offensive can obstruct the purpose of a test when it produces negative feelings, which affect the students' attitudes toward the test, and thus influences their test scores (1996).

The aim of a nursing test is to measure knowledge that is essential to safe nursing practice in the United States. Reading speed, vocabulary ability, or familiarity with cultural practices, which are unrelated to health, should not influence a student's score (Klisch, 1994). It is important that teachers collaborate with each other when developing a nursing exam. Every test should be carefully reviewed by at least two faculty members for items containing language that could offend or be misunderstood. Therefore, an item with overt cultural or gender bias should be rejected. Items referring to events that are common to one culture but not another should also be eliminated. All tests should be carefully edited to remove stereotypical language. In fact, even the most innocent vocabulary can introduce bias into a test (see Figure 2.3). Although offensive, demeaning, or emotionally charged material may not make an item more difficult, it can cause students to become distracted, thus lowering their overall performance (Hambleton & Rodgers, 1995).

Biased Question:
A client who is taking a medication that is a sedative says to a nurse, "I am responsible for the *carpool* tomorrow." Which of these directions should the nurse give to the client?

The term "carpool" could be unfamiliar to individuals for whom English is a second language or for those who live in urban areas and depend on public transportation.

FIGURE 2.3   Example of a culturally biased item

Poorly written test items can introduce structural bias into a test. Items that are grammatically incorrect, ambiguous, or vaguely worded will confuse all students, but they will particularly confuse students for whom English is a second language (ESL students) and learning disabled students (Klisch, 1994). Each question should be succinctly written so that all students have a clear understanding of its meaning the first time it is read. The detailed item development guidelines, which are presented in Chapter 6, "Developing Multiple-Choice Items," will assist you in eliminating bias from your test items.

Following these guidelines will help to keep your exams free from language that can be offensive or introduce bias:

- Avoid use of gender

- Refrain from stereotyping members of a group

- Use references to race, culture, religion, marital status, or sexual orientation only when it pertains to the problem in the question

- Avoid terminology that refers to popular culture and is unrelated to health issues

- Eliminate vocabulary that has a different or unfamiliar meaning to different ethnic groups

Reliability

Test reliability is very important to test developers and users. You would have little confidence in a standardized nursing achievement test that ranked a student in the top five percent last week, but places the same student near the mean this week. Reliability refers to the degree of consistency with which an instrument measures an attribute for a particular group. Reliability is not a property of the test itself; the test is not reliable. Reliability refers to the reproducibility of a set of scores obtained from a particular group, on a particular day, under particular circumstances (Frisbie, 1988). Reliable achievement tests provide consistent results that are reproducible and generalizable. That is, if you were to obtain a second measurement with the same test on the same individual, you would obtain the same result. However, because every measurement contains error, you should expect some variation in test performance. It is highly unlikely that your efforts at obtaining a second measurement would produce precisely the same scores as the first measurement.

Reliability can be quantified by several statistical formulas. These estimates provide a reliability coefficient, or a measure of the amount of variation in test performance. There are several procedures for obtaining a test's reliability estimate. Procedures that are most frequently reported by test analysis software estimate a test's reliability based on the internal consistency of the test. These reliability estimates range from zero to one, with zero indicating no reliability and one indicating perfect reliability. The statistical methods for obtaining reliability estimates are discussed further in Chapter 9, "Establishing Evidence of Reliability and Validity."

The reliability coefficients associated with measures of internal consistency are directly influenced by the spread of scores on the test and the discrimination of the test items (Haladyna, 1997). The larger the score variability or spread of scores, the higher the reliability estimate will be (Linn & Gronlund, 2000). Several factors can introduce error and directly affect the reliability of your multiple-choice classroom tests. Understanding these factors will help you to take appropriate measures to minimize error and maximize the reliability of your classroom tests. Recognizing the influence of these factors on reliability will also enable you to make sensible interpretations of test analysis data.

Quality of the Test Items

The primary requirement for test reliability is that a test has well-constructed items. If the individual test items are clear and focused, they will provide reliable information about student ability or achievement. However, poorly constructed items, which are vague and ambiguous, will be open to a variety of student interpretations and will provide unreliable test results because they will confuse both the high- and low-achievers on a test. The best way to improve classroom test reliability is to improve the quality of individual test items. Chapters 6, "Developing Multiple-Choice Items," and 7, "Writing Critical Thinking Multiple-Choice Items," provide extensive guidelines for developing high quality, multiple-choice items, and Chapter 12, "Instituting Item Banking and Test Development Software," examines how to improve the items based on item analysis data.

Item Difficulty

Test results show little variability when the test items are too easy or too difficult. Tests that are so easy that nearly everyone answers all of the items correctly, or tests that are so difficult that nearly everyone answers all of the items incorrectly, will not identify differences in achievement among students. When the test scores are very similar there is very little score variability. A test with low score variability will have low test reliability (Mehrens & Lehmann, 1973). Thus, presenting students with challenging items within a moderate difficulty range will identify the levels of student achievement and also increase test reliability.

Item Discrimination

Item discrimination is the best indicator of the quality of an item. It identifies the item's ability to differentiate between those who score high and those who score low on a test. If an item is answered correctly by students with high overall test scores and answered incorrectly by students with low overall test scores, the item is said to discriminate, or to differentiate between those who do and those who do not know the material. Highly discriminating items contribute substantially to test score reliability because they distinguish between students of different achievement levels (Frisbie, 1988).

A direct relationship exists between the sum of the discrimination indices on a test and the variance of the test scores—the larger the sum of the discrimination indices, the larger the test variance (Nitko, 1996, p. 314). Therefore, it follows that the higher the average value of a test's item discrimination index, the higher the test's reliability will be (Ebel, 1979, p. 268). A reliable test is made up of items with highly positive discrimination indices. Chapter 10, "Interpreting Test Results," provides further discussion about methods for identifying, interpreting, and improving item discrimination data.

Homogeneity of the Test Content

Measurements of internal consistency estimate a test's reliability by comparing the individual item responses to the total test score. These estimates indicate the extent to which all test items are measuring a single domain (Frisbe, 1998). Therefore, the more consistent the test content is, the higher inter-item consistency and the reliability will be (Anastasi & Urbina, 1997). A test on content, which is narrowly defined, provides a consistent correlation between individual item responses and the total test score, and therefore enhances the test's reliability (Ebel, 1979). For example, in a test that focuses solely on medication calculations, every item is directly related to every other item on the test. That is, the knowledge required to answer each item is very consistent and the total test score directly reflects the student's knowledge of medication calculations.

A test covering a range of content will have heterogeneous items that require different knowledge. For example, in a comprehensive nursing exam, the course objectives are consistent, while areas of content can include clinical knowledge from several areas, including adult health, child health, women's health, and mental health. While all of the questions require nursing expertise, the content knowledge required is very broad. Therefore, the total test scores would not necessarily reflect student knowledge of a particular content area, and the test's reliability will be decreased because the responses to each item will not necessarily correspond to the total test scores.

Many nursing programs utilize an integrated curriculum. Therefore, their exams are built on content areas that vary. It is important to interpret the reliability of this test type with the understanding that the reliability of a comprehensive test will be lower than a test with a narrowly defined content area. A low reliability value can indicate that the test items are measuring a set of skills that are not closely related to each other.

Homogeneity of the Test Group

If most of the items on a test are answered correctly by the majority of the group, the scores will have a small spread, and it will be difficult to distinguish the high achievers from the low ones. When a group has similar abilities, the spread of scores is diminished. Consider the extreme example where everyone receives 100 percent on a test. There is no variability of their test scores. Because everyone has the same score, there is no way to determine how the responses to the individual items compare to the total test scores, and the test has zero reliability. Student nurses usually must meet admission criteria, therefore we should expect a degree of homogeneity in the group. It is important to keep this fact in mind when interpreting the reliability coefficient of a classroom test.

Test Length

A test's reliability increases as the number of items in the test increases. Increasing the number of items in a test decreases the effect of fortuitous responses on the total test score. This is because a longer test provides a more extensive sample of the behavior that is being measured, and it decreases the influence of chance factors, such as guessing (Linn & Gronlund, 2000).

For example, suppose that in order to measure medication calculation ability, you ask students to solve one medication calculation question. The results of this measurement would be highly unreliable. If the question was particularly difficult, most of the students would fail. If you presented an easy problem, most students would pass. As you add questions to the test, the test becomes increasingly more reliable, and you obtain a better estimate of each student's ability. It is important to recognize that the items added to the original test, which increased its length, must have similar statistical properties as the original test. In other words, the additional items must have similar average difficulty and discrimination levels as the items on the original test.

Table 2.5 illustrates how the reliability of a 10-item test with a reliability of 0.3 can be increased by adding items. Note that there is a self-limiting point to adding items to a test to increase its reliability. Thus, the higher the reliability of the original test, the smaller the increase in the reliability will be with the added test length.

TABLE 2.5   The Relation of Test Length to Test Reliability

Number of Items	Test Reliability
10	0.30
20	0.46
40	0.63
80	0.77
160	0.88
320	0.93
640	0.97
∞	1.00

If time constraints limit the number of items that can be included in a test, you may need to administer tests more frequently. There are many reasons why it would be impossible to administer a test consisting of 250 items. Yet, over the course of a semester you probably test your students with at least that many items. The following concept is essential to the meaning of reliable grading: Collect enough data so that you can make reliable decisions about students (Haladyna, 1999).

Number of Examinees

Sample size affects test reliability. Small samples provide a small spread of scores and therefore low variability. It is obvious that the exam results of five students will never be as reliable as the results of 500 students on the same exam. The larger the sample size, the greater the variability of the scores and the higher the reliability of the test.

Speed

Speeded tests are performance tests in which speed plays an important role in determining individual scores. In a speeded test, some of the students do not have time to consider each test item. A power test is one in which there is no time limit, or if there is one it is so generous that the majority of students are able to finish it (Lyman, 1998). If a test score depends on speed, the difference in scores will depend on the difference in the speed with which the individuals answer the questions. An item's position within a speeded test determines whether an individual even gets the opportunity to answer that item. Internal consistency estimates tend to be falsely high on speeded tests because some of the high achieving students reach questions that others do not even have the time to attempt to answer. This increases the mean inter-item correlation and tends to inflate the reliability estimate when internal consistency procedures are used to analyze a speeded test (Thorndike, 1997).

Speed should not be a factor in determining the scores of a classroom test, unless speed is a critical aspect of the test, such as a typing test. Classroom achievement tests should be power tests. All students should be able to comfortably complete the exam in the allotted time. After all, the purpose of an achievement test is to measure student levels of attainment, not to determine how rapidly they can respond to questions. Speeded tests will artificially increase the test's reliability estimate because the score spread will be increased. It is far more preferable to genuinely increase a test's reliability by improving the quality of the test items.

Although there are time constraints imposed on every classroom assessment, it is important to design your exams to allow sufficient time for all students to attempt every item. Presenting a reasonable number of well-developed questions for the allotted test time is the most effective way to increase the reliability of your classroom exams. A general rule-of-thumb is to allow 60 minutes for every 50 multiple-choice items on a test, assuming that all of these items are clear and succinct. Guidelines for developing such items are discussed in Chapters 6, "Developing Multiple-Choice Items," and 7, "Writing Critical Thinking Multiple-Choice Items."

Test Design, Administration, and Scoring

The design of a test and conditions under which students take the test can also affect reliability. If extraneous factors interfere with, or improve, students' ability to select the correct responses, their performance on the test will not reflect their true ability. If the scoring of the test is influenced by extraneous factors, such as cheating, the reliability of the test results again are questionable. These factors must be taken seriously because they introduce measurement error into the testing situation. Chapter 8, "Assembling, Administering, and Scoring a Test," discusses these factors and also provides practical suggestions for minimizing these sources of error in your classroom exams.

Validity

As Figure 2.4 identifies: Although a test must be reliable to be valid, a reliable test is not always valid. A test can have high reliability and yet not really measure anything of importance; or it can fail to be an appropriate measure for a particular use (Burns & Grove, 1997). Therefore, we can have reliable measures that provide the wrong information.

A test can be reliable without being valid.

HOWEVER

A test cannot be valid unless it is reliable.

FIGURE 2.4   Reliability requirement for validity

"Validity is the most fundamental consideration in developing and evaluating tests" (AERA et al., 1999, p. 9). Validity is not a property of the test itself. It refers to the appropriateness of the interpretation of the test scores—the extent of the evidence that exists to justify the inferences we make based on the results of the test. A test can have substantial evidence of validity for one interpretation and not for another. For example, an exam can have considerable evidence of validity for interpretations related to acceptance into a city's police department; while the same exam can be of no use for admission to the same city's fire department. This is a perfect example of why you cannot use an exam with validity evidence, which supports its use to assess theoretical nursing knowledge, to also assess a construct such as critical thinking—unless you can collect validity evidence to justify the test's use to measure critical thinking.

Validity does not exist on an all-or-none basis. A test is always valid to some degree—high, moderate, or weak in a particular situation with a particular sample. Validity is a matter of judgment—there are no fixed rules for deciding what is meant by high, moderate, or weak validity. Skill in making these judgments is based on test validation, and it develops with experience in dealing with tests (Lyman, 1998). Test validation is defined as the process of collecting evidence to establish that the inferences, which are made based on the test results, are appropriate. One of the basics to this skill development is a clear understanding of the types of evidence that establish validity:

- content-related evidence

- construct-related evidence

- criterion-related evidence

In the traditional approach to establishing validity, there were three classifications: content validity, construct validity, and criterion-related validity. Today, however, validity is not viewed as three separate types. The 1985 edition of the *Standards for Educational and Psychological Testing* identifies validity as a unitary concept that includes each of the categories as evidence of validity. Content-related evidence, criterion-related evidence, and construct-related evidence are interrelated; ideal validation includes several types of evidence, spanning all three of the traditional categories (AERA, p. 9). This approach emphasizes that validity is not an all-or-none proposition. It is a matter of degree and involves the judgment that you make after considering all of the accumulated evidence.

The most recent edition of the *Standards for Educational and Psychological Testing* refers to types of validity evidence rather than to distinct types of validity. In fact, in an attempt to emphasize that validation is a process of collecting a variety of evidence to support a proposed interpretation of a test, this edition does not follow the traditional nomenclature. Rather, it outlines the various sources of evidence that can be used for evaluating the proposed interpretation of a test's score for a particular purpose (AERA et al., 1999, p. 11).

When reviewing the different types of validity evidence, it is essential to keep the unitary nature of validity in mind. Types of validity evidence do not exist exclusively or separately. The categories overlap; all categories are essential to a unitary concept of validity. Evidence from each one may be needed when attempting to validate the interpretations of a test scores.

Content-Related Evidence of Validity

Content-related evidence represents the degree to which the items on a test reflect a course's content domain. Content-related validity is nonstatistical (Lyman, 1998); it cannot be objectively quantified with a number. Rather, the documentation of content-related evidence of validity begins with test development and is established by a detailed examination of the test content. The more closely related a test is to its blueprint, the higher the content validity will be. If a test has content-related evidence of validity, then we can use the test results to make a judgment about the person's knowledge within that specific content domain.

A well-constructed test measures every important aspect of a course, including the subject matter and the course objectives (Anastasi & Urbina, 1997). Because a test measures only a sample of a domain, representativeness is the key issue in content validation. No aspect of a course should be under- or over-represented. The validity of the inferences based on the test results is dependent upon how well the test sample represents the domain being tested (Worthen, Borg, & White, 1993, p.182). A blueprint establishes content-related evidence of validity by ensuring that a test provides a representative sampling of the objectives and content domain of a course. Chapter 5, "Implementing Systematic Test Development," presents detailed guidelines for developing blueprints for your classroom tests.

Content-related evidence of validity is a central concern during test development (AERA et al., 1985, p. 11). Tests that provide content valid results are produced with careful planning. Standardized tests utilize a national panel of experts in the field being measured to establish evidence of their content-related validity. When you develop a classroom test, you do not have access to a panel of experts. However, you can strengthen the evidence for the validity of your tests by developing the tests from a blueprint at the course's outset and by following the steps for enhancing content-related evidence of test validity (Figure 2.5).

Construct-Related Evidence of Validity

A construct is an unobservable characteristic of an individual that cannot be measured directly, such as intelligence, creativity, and critical thinking. When we desire to use a test to measure an unobservable characteristic, we must require that the test have construct-related evidence of validity. Construct validation involves the collection of evidence, which supports the assertion that a test measures a construct by measuring the observable behaviors, which demonstrate the construct as defined by the test developer (Worthen, Borg, & White, 1993, p. 187). Content-related and criterion-related evidence can also support construct interpretation.

- State objectives in performance terms

- Identify learning outcomes

- Define the domain to be measured

- Prepare a detailed blueprint

- Write items to fit the blueprint

- Select a representative sample of items for the test

- Ask colleagues to review your blueprint and items

- Provide adequate time for test completion

- Review item and test analysis

- Use the test only for its intended purpose

FIGURE 2.5 Steps for enhancing content-related evidence of test validity

Construct validation begins with test development, and it continues until the evidence establishes that there is a relationship between the test scores and the construct. For example, a test claiming to measure critical thinking would require construct validation. First, a detailed definition of the construct of critical thinking, which is derived from psychological theory, prior research, or systematic observation and analyses of the behavior domain, must be developed (Anastasi & Urbina, 1997, p. 138). The definition should delineate the aspects of the construct that are to be represented in the test. Then, the objectives and learning outcomes that correlate with the definition must be specified. Once this is completed, the test is blueprinted, and items are developed, which require students to demonstrate the behaviors that define the construct of critical thinking.

A variety of methods can be used to collect data to establish construct-related evidence for a new critical thinking test. These methods include the following:

- Obtaining intercorrelations of test items to provide evidence of item homogeneity, which supports the assertion that the new test is measuring one construct (AERA et al., 1999, p. 13).

- Correlating the score on the new critical thinking test with scores from other instruments, which have demonstrated ability to measure critical thinking. A positive correlation would support the identification of critical thinking in the new test (AERA et al. 1999, p. 13).

- Questioning the takers of the new test about their thinking strategies by asking them to think aloud about their mental processes as they answer the questions. This supports the definition of the construct and provides evidence of the cognitive processes involved within the construct (AERA et al., 1999, p. 12).

- Asking experts in the area of critical thinking to judge the relationship of the items on the test with the construct of critical thinking (AERA et al., 1999, p. 11) to verify that the items are measuring the construct.

A multitude of commercially prepared exams maintain that they assess critical thinking. It is very important for you to be an informed consumer when purchasing one of these exams to administer to your students. A variety of evidence must be collected in order to establish that a test is measuring the construct it purports to measure. When reviewing a standardized exam that claims to measure critical thinking, it is important to closely examine its reliability evidence and to ask the following questions:

- What is the definition of critical thinking?

- What are the objectives of the test?

- What are the learning outcomes on which the questions are based?

- What is the structure of the test's blueprint?

You should expect the test developer to answer these questions and provide information about the experts who were involved at every level of the test development process. The developer should also provide you with data about the test's reliability. In addition, you should also expect the developer to report the evidence that they have accumulated to support the validity of the proposed interpretations of the test. If the answers to these questions are unavailable or unclear, select another test.

One of the goals of this book is to provide a framework for faculty to develop multiple-choice items that assess critical thinking. Ask the same questions that you would ask when evaluating a standardized test. Once these questions are addressed, you can write multiple-choice items to measure the behaviors that provide evidence of critical thinking abilities. Chapters 4, "Assessing Critical Thinking," and 7, "Writing Critical Thinking Multiple-Choice Items," discuss the development of multiple-choice test items that measure critical thinking abilities in greater detail.

Criterion-Related Evidence of Validity

Criterion-related evidence of validity demonstrates that test scores are systematically related to one or more outcome criteria (AERA et al., 1985, p. 11). The focus of a study on predictive evidence is to determine how valid a test is at predicting a second measure of performance—the criteria. A study of concurrent evidence, however, is concerned with estimating present performance when compared to the criterion. The key question with criterion-related validity is: "How accurately do test scores estimate criterion performance?" (AERA et al., 1999, p. 14).

As Lyman explains, concurrent and predictive evidence differ only in their time sequence. Both test scores and criterion values are obtained at about the same time with concurrent validity. However, in predictive validity, there is a time lapse between testing and obtaining the criterion values. When criterion-related evidence is high, the test can be used to estimate performance on the criterion (1998).

If you are using a test score to predict future performance, you must be concerned with determining the degree of the relationship between the test and the criterion (the future performance). Support of criterion validity must include empirical evidence on the comparison between test performance and performance of the criterion (Rudner, 1994). Many tests are currently being marketed that claim to predict student success on the NCLEX. When evaluating these predictor exams, it is important for you to determine how they have established criterion-related evidence of validity. You should be able to answer this question: How does the test predict the performance of the students on NCLEX? The predictor test should compare an individual's test scores to NCLEX pass/fail status, in order to provide a basis for predicting the likelihood of passing or failing NCLEX based on the score on the predictor test.

Beware of exams claiming to have an extremely high accuracy rate for predicting the passing rate on the NCLEX exam. Look closely at their statistics. For example, if a company says that it can predict NCLEX success with a 98 percent accuracy rate, what test score does a student need to obtain to qualify for the passing prediction? If, for example, a test predicts success for students who answer more than 90 percent of the test questions correctly, what is the test really predicting? When fewer than 20 percent of a group taking a test are predicted to pass, of what use is the prediction? A conservative estimate of the students who will pass is a safe approach to predicting NCLEX outcomes. When a company predicts that 20 percent of a group of students will pass, does the company also predict how many will fail? Find out how accurate the test is at predicting students who will fail NCLEX. The prediction of failure is much more useful—particularly if the test report delineates the students' weaknesses and proposes a plan for remediation.

Most faculty can accurately identify the top 20 percent of their students, based on their history of classroom test results. In addition, 84.8 percent of first time, U.S.-educated candidates passed the NCLEX in 1999 (Yocum & White, 1999, p. 30). A test predicting the success of a very small number of students—who will obviously pass—is really predicting nothing at all!

Face Validity

Face validity is not validity in the technical sense; it refers to what a test appears to measure, and not what it actually measures. Face validity means that the appearance of the test coincides with its use (Popham, 1999). While actual validity is far more important than face validity, face validity is still desirable. A test needs face validity so that it *appears* valid to the test consumer. Face validity also helps to keep the motivation of the test takers high—students seem to try harder when a test appears to be reasonable and fair (Lyman, 1998). In fact, a test that appears irrelevant or inappropriate will create a diversion and can even result in poor cooperation from the test takers (Anastasi & Urbina, 1997). Thus, students will respond positively to tests that represent the content and objectives of the course. Tests which are perceived as unrelated to course content can distract students and therefore decrease the test's reliability.

It is helpful for a test to have face validity, as long as it has demonstrated evidence of actual validity (Polit & Hungler, 1999). Face validity by itself never provides sufficient basis on which to establish validity; the mere appearance of validity is not adequate to establish evidence of validity. We must still establish evidence that enables us to be confident in the decisions we make based on the test's scores.

Usually when you establish evidence of validity for an interpretation of test scores, face validity is also established. Poor test item construction is a primary cause of inadequate face validity. Thus, nursing exams should refer to nursing situations. Developing an exam blueprint and including a nurse and a client in the questions will add to the face validity of your nursing exams. Sharing the blueprint with the students before the test will alert them about what to expect on the test, and will also increase their perception of the test as a valid measurement.

Basic Test Statistics

Test analysis is a powerful tool that you can use to increase the quality of your classroom exams and your confidence in the decisions you make based on the test results. In addition, item analysis is an invaluable guide for improving the reliability and validity of future tests by directing the improvement of the individual test items. Before you can analyze test and item data and correctly interpret their meanings, it is important that you understand the basic concepts of test statistics. Appendix A, "Basic Test Statistics," provides a brief reference guide to help familiarize you with the terms related to test and item analysis, which are used throughout the book. Each of these definitions are examined in greater detail in Chapters 10, "Interpreting Test Results," and 12, "Instituting Item Banking and Test Development Software," where you will find in-depth discussions on test and item analysis.

Summary

Assessment procedures do not make decisions about students, teachers make decisions about students. In order to develop procedures that ensure fair decisions, it is important to have a clear understanding of the principles of assessment. This chapter presents an overview of the terminology that is fundamental to a thorough understanding of the concepts underlying valid and reliable assessment procedures. Many of these concepts are explained in greater detail in subsequent chapters. This book explores every aspect of the assessment process and offers guidelines for the development of valid and reliable multiple-choice exams that are an integral component of a plan for the systematic assessment of learning outcomes. An understanding of the "Language of Assessment" is the basic requirement for establishing a comprehensive assessment plan.

3 Developing Instructional Objectives

*"You tell me, and I forget. You teach me, and I remember.
You involve me, and I learn."*

—Benjamin Franklin

Before you can develop a plan for the assessment of outcomes, you must first determine what the outcomes will be. Learning outcomes are derived from the objectives for an instructional course. While objectives clarify the instructional destination of an educational experience for both the teacher and the students, outcomes are the behaviors that represent the achievement of those objectives.

The first step in developing an assessment plan is to identify the course objectives. These objectives set the stage for effective planning, teaching, and assessment by specifying what a student should know and be able to do at the end of an instructional course (Weimer, 1996). However, educators often focus on what material should be included in a course before identifying what knowledge and skills they want students to develop. Identifying the objectives and outcomes as the initial step in planning guides the instructional and assessment processes for a course and also provides the framework for developing valid and reliable measurement instruments, including multiple-choice exams.

Students are much more likely to succeed if they understand what is expected of them right from the outset of an educational experience. Establishing outcomes during the initial phase of course preparation will compel you to identify your learning expectations in language that explicitly communicates your intent to students. Clearly-defined learning objectives steer efficient course planning. In addition, they also guide the selection of teaching and learning activities, direct the development of measurement instruments, and empower students to take charge of their own learning to meet your expectations, thereby increasing the validity of your assessment plan.

Role of Objectives

Objectives guide the instructional process by synchronizing the planning and implementation of teaching, learning, and assessment activities, thereby focusing on the outcomes teachers want students to achieve. Unfortunately, course preparation too often involves planning for the content and teaching activities without a clear definition of what student outcomes are desired. This approach can lead to instructional methods and assessments that focus on knowledge acquisition rather than on higher-level learning outcomes.

If students are expected to achieve the outcomes of a course, they must be provided with appropriate opportunities to learn what they need to learn (Huba & Freed, 2000). Instructional objectives require teachers to provide students with the kinds of experiences that facilitate the attainment of the objectives. When objectives are determined at the beginning of a course, they provide direction to the teacher for selection of the instructional activities that promote achievement of the desired behaviors (Gronlund, 2000). For example, a course objective requiring a student to utilize critical thinking necessitates that the teacher select learning experiences and assessment activities that require the ability to think critically.

With today's advancing technology, the need for developing innovative approaches to facilitate learning is paramount. The pervasive nature of the Internet and the rapid progression of distance learning mandates that teachers develop creative teaching modalities and learning opportunities to meet learner preferences. In this atmosphere of self-directed learning, instructional objectives are assuming an ever increasing role as the basis for meeting the diverse needs of learners.

When students are aware of what is required of them from the beginning of a course, they are given responsibility for their own learning and the opportunity to direct their activities toward achieving the required outcomes (Reilly & Oermann, 1990). Self-direction is facilitated when an individual learner has the ability to decide how to meet a course's objectives by selecting from a variety of teaching/learning strategies that are designed to accommodate diverse individual learning styles.

Instructional objectives and learning outcomes also play a crucial role as the basis for valid measurement instruments by providing the framework on which a test blueprint is based. As Chapter 5, "Implementing Systematic Test Development," describes in detail, the blueprint directs the content of the test. In addition to shaping the blueprint, the objectives guide the development of the test items. Chapters 6, "Developing Multiple-Choice Items," and Chapter 7, "Writing Critical Thinking Multiple-Choice Items," illustrate how multiple-choice items evolve from the learning outcomes. The most important role of the instructional objectives is to increase the validity of assessments. When student achievement is measured with instruments that are based on instructional outcomes, fairness is assured.

Focus of Instructional Objectives

What is the most effective way to state an instructional objective? Figure 3.1 presents two different approaches for defining one of the desired outcomes for a hypothetical course in the fundamentals of nursing care.

Teacher-Focused: To demonstrate to students how to safely perform basic nursing procedures.

Learner-Focused: The student will demonstrate safe performance of basic nursing procedures.

FIGURE 3.1 Teacher-focused versus learner-focused instructional objectives

In a teacher-focused objective, the attention is centered on the teaching activity. Teaching is an end in itself; learning is not a criteria. The objective, in effect, is met once the teaching has taken place, no matter if the teaching is effective. This approach to instruction focuses on transmitting information and explains the all-too-common teacher lament, "I don't understand why the students do not know that material. I covered it in class."

In a learner-focused objective, the concern is focused on the learning that occurs in relation to the teaching that is taking place. Stating instructional objectives in terms of the required student achievement shifts the focus of the educational experience from transmitting volumes of information to providing learning experiences that foster attainment of those outcomes. Teaching thus becomes a means to an outcome, rather than an end in itself.

Learner-focused objectives require teachers to examine their teaching strategies and to develop creative methods that facilitate student learning. With this approach, if students do not achieve the desired outcomes, the first question that a teacher must ask is, "Were the instructional experiences appropriate?"

It is important to recognize that teachers who do not consciously identify instructional objectives are most likely operating on teacher-focused goals. When the main objective of classroom instruction is to *cover the material*, without concern for developing strategies to meet student needs, the goals are teacher-focused and the approach usually is a didactic one. Although this instructional method can require students to think logically, it does not encourage critical thinking. While the lecture approach to teaching is the easiest one for the teacher, it can be the least beneficial for the students.

Huba and Freed (2000, pp. 9–15) identify the four following fundamental requirements for the development of effective learner-focused assessment:

1. *Formulate statements of intended learning outcomes.* The first step is to describe the intentions for what students should know, understand, and be able to do with their knowledge when they graduate.

2. *Develop or select assessment measures.* In order to measure whether the intended outcomes are achieved, data-gathering measures must be utilized. Designing these measures forces the teacher to understand thoroughly what is really meant by the intended learning outcomes.

3. *Create experiences leading to the outcomes.* If students are expected to achieve the intended outcomes, they must be provided with appropriate opportunities to achieve those outcomes.

4. *Discuss and use assessment results to improve learning.* Discussions must take place in order to use assessment data for the improvement of learning. These discussions should occur between faculty and students and among the faculty as well in order to gain insights into the learning that is occurring.

Taxonomies

A taxonomy is a system that describes, identifies, and classifies groups. In education, taxonomies classify three domains of learning—cognitive, affective, and psychomotor. In 1956, the *Taxonomy of Educational Objectives,* edited by Benjamin Bloom, was published. Popularly referred to as *Bloom's Taxonomy,* this well known resource for the development of instructional objectives and test items initially covered only the cognitive domain of learning. Subsequent editions, however, deal with the affective and psychomotor learning domains as well.

Bloom's taxonomy classifies three domains of learning:

- *Cognitive*   Concerned with intellectual objectives. Bloom describes this domain as the central point of the work of most test development; it deals with knowledge and the development of intellectual abilities and skills (p. 7).

- *Affective*   Objectives in this domain describe interests, attitudes, and values (p. 7). In nursing education, this domain relates to how these characteristics impact on the practice of nursing.

- *Psychomotor*   Bloom refers to this domain as the manipulative or motor-skill area (p. 7). This domain is concerned with physical movements that require coordination. Oermann (1990) identifies that psychomotor skills have a cognitive aspect, which involves understanding the principles underlying each skill, and an affective dimension, which is concerned with a nurse's values and attitudes while performing a skill.

Taxonomies relate to educational goals and are especially useful for establishing objectives and developing test items. Each domain is organized by levels of increasing complexity within the domain category. The cognitive domain, for example, includes the levels of knowledge, comprehension, application, and analysis. The levels build on each other with knowledge being the lowest level. The cognitive domain is particularly applicable to multiple-choice test development. In nursing, multiple-choice items are most effective when written at the application and analysis levels. In fact, these are the cognitive levels at which multiple-choice items are written for the NCLEX (National Council of State Boards of Nursing [NCSBN], 1998, p. 3). These cognitive levels can be described as follows:

- *Knowledge*   Requires the recall of previously learned material, it refers to the simple remembrance of a fact, concept, theory, or principle. A learner is expected to remember information exactly as it is presented in a textbook or from a classroom lecture.

- *Comprehension*   Refers to the ability to grasp the meaning of material. Comprehension is demonstrated by translating material from one form to another. A learner is expected to translate facts, to interpret the importance of the information, to take in information and *give it back* in another way, and to make predictions based on understanding.

- *Application*   Requires the utilization of learned material in new and concrete situations. Application calls for a student to apply concepts, laws, methods, phenomena, principles, procedures, rules, and theories in unique real-life situations.

- *Analysis*   Involves the ability to break down material into its component parts so that its organizational structure can be understood. The ability to analyze requires a student to breakdown information, view the relationships among the parts, recognize the effects, and understand the meaning of the information.

Taxonomies provide a useful framework for the development of objectives that accurately reflect the levels of learning. The taxonomy for each of the previous domains begins with its basic skills and progresses to its more complex abilities. Referring to a taxonomy assures you that important categories of learning are not overlooked. Linn and Gronlund suggest that a taxonomy be used as an aid in the development of your own unique list of objectives (2000). Once your objectives are established, a taxonomy is also valuable in the design of test questions to accommodate your objectives.

Several taxonomies have been developed—each with its own classification scheme. Nitko (1996) presents a general discussion of several taxonomies. He cautions the user of a taxonomy to remember that "1) thinking skills may not be hierarchical and 2) student performance of complex tasks involves using several thinking skills at the same time" (p. 28).

Taxonomies can be useful as a guide in the development of a comprehensive list of high quality objectives. However, it is counterproductive to use a taxonomy as a rigid rule book for developing objectives or test questions.

Stating Instructional Objectives

Unless students are well informed about assessment criteria, they are placed in a no-win situation. However, by stating the instructional objectives in terms of the behaviors you expect from your students, you give them the direction they need to succeed. A meaningful objective communicates desired outcome behavior of the learner *exactly* as you understand it. Therefore, if another teacher uses your objective and their student outcomes are consistent with your expectations, then you have communicated the objective in a meaningful way (Mager, 1962).

Specific Objectives

Methods for writing instructional objectives include general and specific formats. A highly specific format delineates student outcomes in very specific terms. Linn and Gronlund describe how specific objectives can be further defined by a list of specific tasks. These tasks can then be taught and tested sequentially. While this process can clearly define student outcomes, it tends to overemphasize low-level skills and factual knowledge, and also stresses simple learning outcomes (2000, p. 56). Narrowly focused specific objectives also raise a concern that students can be led to focus only on limited information, thus excluding important concepts.

McMillan identifies behavior, audience (learner), criterion, and condition as the components of highly precise objectives (1997, p. 25). Figure 3.2 is an example of a highly specific objective that identifies these components.

Within twenty minutes in the learning laboratory (condition), the student (learner) will obtain (behavior) an apical pulse on a volunteer that is accurate to within three beats per minute (criterion).

FIGURE 3.2   An example of a specific instructional objective

Highly specific objectives clearly indicate the behaviors that a student must demonstrate to achieve the objective. However, the degree of specificity inherent in these objectives makes them unwieldy. In a complex discipline such as nursing, faculty would certainly have to develop extensive lists of specific objectives in order to include every course outcome. In addition, these objectives are very confining because they severely limit a teacher's ability to modify the instructional approach. McMillan suggests that it is better to focus your objectives on units of instruction rather than on daily lesson plans because "writing objectives that are too specific results in long lists of minutia that are too time consuming to monitor and manage" (1997, p. 26).

General Objectives

Oermann and Gaberson suggest that a general format is preferred over a specific format for writing objectives in a complex area of study, such as nursing. In fact, they describe a format for writing general objectives that is open-ended—it identifies the expected learning outcomes, but does not prescribe particular learning conditions or assessment strategies. The format consists of a learner, a behavior, and the content (1998, p. 9). Figure 3.3 restates the specific objective (referred to in Figure 3.2) as a general objective.

The student (learner) will demonstrate (behavior) safe performance of basic nursing procedures (content).

FIGURE 3.3   An example of a specific objective restated as general objective

This general objective format accommodates the development of higher-order thinking skills and leaves room for creativity in achieving and assessing the prescribed outcomes (Reilly & Oermann, 1990).

Gronlund (2000) suggests that stating the general learning objective first, and then listing a representative sample of learning outcomes clarifies for the student what is acceptable to the teacher as evidence for attaining the objective. When this approach is used, it is acceptable to use words that are open to broad interpretation in a general learning objective, because they are followed by specific statements of measurable behaviors, or learning outcomes, describing what a learner should be doing as evidence that the objective is attained (Mager, 1962). Using a word such as *comprehend* is suitable for a general objective because it is clarified by the learning outcomes so that the learner knows exactly what behavior indicates the ability to comprehend.

Learning Outcomes

Consider the general objective shown in Figure 3.3. Although it is learner-focused, it is very general and does not clearly specify what behaviors a student must demonstrate in order to confirm attainment of the objective. In order to provide a basis for student assessment, the behaviors acceptable as evidence of the attainment of a general objective must be identified. Figure 3.4 provides an example of the learning outcomes for the student-focused general instructional objective in Figure 3.3.

The student will demonstrate safe performance of basic nursing procedures:

Identifies the rationale for the procedure.

Acknowledges the impact of the procedure on the client.

Describes the steps of the procedure.

Explains the procedure to the client.

Selects the appropriate equipment for the procedure.

Performs the procedure with a predetermined degree of accuracy.

Maintains appropriate aseptic technique during the procedure.

Interprets client responses to the procedure.

Communicates the results of the procedure appropriately.

Provides client follow-up based on the results of the procedure.

FIGURE 3.4   An example of a general objective with its learning outcomes

The general learning objective requires that a student safely perform basic nursing procedures. However, what does *safely perform basic nursing procedures* actually mean? While the general objective is very broad, the learning outcomes are specific behaviors. When considered together, the learning outcomes clarify the general objective by providing an operational definition for what a teacher regards as safe performance of basic nursing procedures.

Note that each learning outcome begins with a *clarifying* verb—a verb that denotes a behavior that can be measured. Clarifying verbs operationalize the general objective. A student who successfully demonstrates these behaviors—at a performance level predetermined by the teacher—would meet the criteria for safe performance of basic nursing procedures.

Gronlund (2000) suggests that while it is important to keep the learning outcomes specific, it is also important to keep them free of specific content so that they can be applied across all units of study in a course. Consider the objective in Figure 3.4. It does not specify which procedures the student must safely perform; the learning outcomes are applicable to all basic nursing procedures.

When stated without specific content, learning outcomes can be applied for establishing evidence of mastery of the learning tasks required for many procedures. For example, *identify the rationale for the procedure* applies to all nursing procedures, while *describe the steps of the procedure* requires that a checklist is developed for each procedure. This approach provides consistency across content for both student and teacher. It requires that a teacher carefully consider the universal requirements for safety across nursing procedures. In addition, it allows for individualization of the requirements for each procedure. It also reinforces the concepts that principles often apply across procedures, while special consideration must be made for individual situations.

One way that you can determine if a person is knowledgeable of something is to observe the individual's behavior. As Mager states, ". . . the most important characteristic of a useful objective is that it identifies the kind of performance that will be accepted as evidence that the learner has achieved the objective" (1962, p. 13). The goal is to communicate your objectives so that they are not subject to misinterpretation. The challenge is to write your objectives at an appropriate level of generality—not so narrow that they are impossible to manage and not so general that they provide little guidance for instruction (McMillan, 1997, p. 26). Table 3.1 provides examples of the verbs used in general objectives and verbs that are used in the learning outcomes to clarify the meaning of an objective.

TABLE 3.1   General and Clarifying Verbs

General Objective Verbs	Clarifying Outcome Verbs		
Apply	Acknowledge	Identify	Tell
Appreciate	Allot	Illustrate	Utilize
Believe	Appoint	Indicate	
Clarify	Arrange	Itemize	
Consider	Assign	Label	
Comprehend	Calculate	List	
Deduce	Categorize	Measure	
Grasp	Choose	Name	
Infer	Cite	Outline	
Interpret	Classify	Perform	
Know	Define	Predict	
Observe	Delegate	Provide	
Recognize	Denote	Recite	
Respect	Describe	Rephrase	
Think	Diagram	Report	
Understand	Differentiate	Select	
Value	Discuss	Specify	
	Enumerate	State	
	Explain	Stipulate	

A list of instructional objectives for a course usually includes objectives that address the mastery of the minimal essentials, as well as objectives that focus on development beyond the minimum level (Gronlund, 2000). Developing objectives and measuring these two different levels require two different sets of criteria. In order to assure that the objectives form a valid basis for the development of multiple-choice items, you must have a clear understanding of the two levels.

Mastery Level Objectives

At the mastery level the domain of learning tasks is limited and can be clearly defined (Gronlund, 1973). Learning outcomes, which measure mastery, are usually outcomes that we can expect all students to master at a minimum level of competence. A teacher must decide which objectives must be mastered and must identify the criteria for mastery.

Objectives at the mastery level are designed to establish a specified minimum performance level, which establishes mastery. Determining a minimum mastery level is an arbitrary process because there is little empirical evidence that supports a specific minimum level. For example, Gronlund (1973) suggests teachers set the level at 85 percent correct for multiple-choice tests, and then adjust the rate as needed. This criterion means that students are required to obtain a score of 85 percent correct to attain mastery. It does not mean that 85 percent of the students will attain mastery. In fact, nursing students are a select group of students—all of them should be able to succeed. As Reilly and Oermann point out, studies of aptitude distribution indicate that 95 percent of students have the potential to achieve mastery of an objective. They note that the teaching-learning experience is most successful when teachers adopt the attitude that all but a possible few students—those who have a particular disability for a particular type of learning—have the potential for success. This attitude fosters the development of teaching and learning strategies that consider and accommodate the individual differences among learners. Teachers who incorporate these strategies are thus able to diagnose student needs and provide appropriate support services to assist all students in achieving mastery (1990).

Gronlund notes that some objectives require a higher level of achievement to establish mastery of safe performance than others (1973). Safety is certainly a concern that nursing faculty must consider when setting mastery levels for nursing procedures such as medication administration. For example, many nursing programs require students to attain a score of 90 to 100 percent correct on a math calculation exam before allowing them to give medications.

No matter what level is set for mastery attainment, teachers must be ready to accept the challenge presented by Reilly and Oermann: To develop strategies to meet the needs of all students in achieving mastery of learning (1990). The best approach for defining mastery is to first establish a consensus among the nursing faculty for the minimum level of mastery for safe nursing practice. Teachers can then provide instructional activities that foster mastery, and finally, adjust the level required for evidence of mastery as needed.

Developmental Level Objectives

Developmental learning is learning beyond the mastery level. While mastery level objectives are directed at the tasks to be performed, developmental-level objectives emphasize progress toward goals. The skills and abilities associated with developmental learning are continuously developing throughout life (Nitko, 1996). Students cannot be expected to fully achieve these objectives during a course of study—each objective represents a goal to work toward. Because each objective at this level represents a large number of specific behaviors, all we can do when defining the objective is to list a reasonable sample of the defining behaviors as learning outcomes (Gronlund, 2000).

Gronlund (1973) explains that outcomes at the developmental level represent the progress made toward attaining the objective:

> It would be impossible to identify all of the behaviors involved in such a complex pattern of response. Even if we could, the measurement of each specific behavior would not be the same as measuring the integrated response pattern. Thus, we need to focus on the types of student performance that are most indicative of progress toward the objectives at that particular level of instruction (p. 17).

Consider the ability to apply the nursing process. This ability certainly represents developmental learning. It requires the development of skills that progress from novice to expert. An example of a specific objective designed to address the ability to apply the nursing process is shown in Figure 3.5.

Specific Nursing Process Objective

Given an assignment to care for an acutely ill client (condition), the student (learner) will

- Collect (behavior) data from at least two sources (criteria).

- Identify (behavior) two nursing diagnoses based on the data (criteria).

- Implement (behavior) two interventions to address each diagnoses (criteria).

- Cite (behavior) two findings that indicate success or failure for each intervention (criteria).

FIGURE 3.5   A nursing process specific objective

The drawbacks for using the specific format for developmental-level learning objectives is evident. This nursing process specific objective is far too narrow and leaves no leeway for teaching, learning, or assessment. Nor does it represent the concept of progress toward a goal. Figure 3.6 restates this objective in a general format.

The student (learner) will apply (behavior) the nursing process in selected health care situations (content).

FIGURE 3.6   A nursing process specific objective restated as a general objective

This objective does not restrict the instructional process because it does not specify the number of sources, diagnoses, interventions, or evaluation findings. However, it does not provide adequate guidance for the instructional process. Figure 3.7 goes further to clarify this objective by specifying the learning outcomes.

---

2. Applies the nursing process in selected health care situations:

2.1   Collects assessment data.

2.2   Identifies nursing diagnoses based on assessment.

2.3   Plans interventions based on analysis of data.

2.4   Maintains safety when implementing nursing plan.

2.5   Adapts plan to individual situations.

2.6   Distinguishes success or failure of plan based on subjective and objective data.

FIGURE 3.7   A nursing process general objective with learning outcomes

The general objective with learning outcomes approach is clearly the most effective strategy for stating objectives related to developmental-level learning. The list of learning outcomes in Figure 3.7 serves to operationalize the general objective by specifying a sample of behaviors, which demonstrate the application of the nursing process. This list of learning outcomes is also free of specific course content—achievement of the objective *applies the nursing process* can be demonstrated across the course content. In addition, the outcomes can apply to students who have different levels of expertise in their progress toward applying the nursing process. Refer to Table 3.2 for a comparison of mastery and developmental learning objectives.

TABLE 3.2   Comparison of Mastery-Level and Developmental-Level Learning Objectives

Mastery Learning Objectives	Developmental Learning Objectives
Well-defined performance domain	Broad domain of related performances
Task oriented	Goal oriented
Focus on knowledge outcomes	Focus on complex achievements
Identify minimum skills	Identify abilities that continuously develop through life
Identify specific performance tasks	Identify a representative sample of performance
Measure attainable abilities	Measure the degree of achievement
Assess narrowly defined skill set	Assess progress toward an ultimate goal

Intermediate Objectives

The objective shown in Figure 3.7 follows the two-step process proposed by Linn and Gronlund (2000):

1. *Each general instructional objective should encompass a readily definable domain of student responses.*   Each general objective should begin with a general verb (for example, knows, understands, applies), consist of only one objective, and be content-free. Typically, eight to twelve general objectives per course will suffice.

2. *List beneath each general instructional objective a representative sample of specific learning outcomes stated in terms of student performance.*   Each learning outcome should begin with an action verb (for example, identifies, describes), be relevant to the general instructional objective, and be relatively free of course content so that it can be applied across various units of study (p. 71).

Linn and Gronlund (2000) describe this as an intermediate framework for developing objectives—one that is not so specific that it fractionalizes learning, nor so general that it fails to communicate instructional intent (p. 70). This framework is particularly suitable for nursing curricula, where many abilities build on each other and are developed over time.

Figure 3.8 presents a template for the development of intermediate objectives for a nursing program. Note that the verb in the general instructional objective represents higher-order cognitive thinking—application. Another aspect of higher-order thinking—analysis—is subsumed in the learning outcomes. Lower-level thinking—knowledge and comprehension—is included in the specific learning outcomes. An application ability requires ability at all levels of cognitive ability. If you cannot define a concept, it is unlikely that you will be able to apply it.

---

1. Applies [Nursing Theory, Communication Skills, Therapeutic Nursing Care, etc.]

1.1   Defines

1.2   Infers

1.3   Interprets

1.4   Analyzes

1.5   Uses

1.6   Evaluates

FIGURE 3.8   Template for intermediate level nursing objectives

This template assumes that the construct being measured has been defined, and the instructional objectives and learning outcomes are derived directly from that definition. The specific verbs for the general objective and learning outcomes should be selected to measure the defined construct. This example illustrates how objectives can be developed to address the levels of cognitive ability across levels and content within a nursing program. A further discussion of the challenges associated with creating objectives for higher-order thinking, particularly critical thinking at the developmental level, is addressed in Chapter 4, "Assessing Critical Thinking."

NUMBER OF OBJECTIVES   Linn and Gronlund's (2000) description of the process of objective development draws attention to a question that nursing faculty frequently ask: "How many objectives should a course have?" While Linn and Gronlund suggest that eight to twelve objectives will suffice (p. 66), there is no hard and fast rule. However, writing your objectives using the intermediate framework previously described will certainly enable you to keep your list manageable. If your objectives apply across content areas, you can apply the outcomes to each unit of study within your course. It is important that you list the abilities you want students to have at a course's end, translate those abilities into general instructional objectives, develop your learning outcomes to operationalize the instructional objectives, and keep the objectives and outcomes content free.

If you are concerned with meeting the accreditation criteria of the NLNAC, I suggest that you include in each of your nursing courses an intermediate-level objective with learning outcomes that address each of the required outcomes; therapeutic nursing interventions, communication, and critical thinking. These objectives will form the basis for a systematic plan for evaluation of the required outcomes. If your objectives are written according to an intermediate framework, the same objective can be used in every course and each of its learning outcomes, instructional activities, and assessment criteria can be developed to show progress in the developmental learning associated with the required outcomes.

Chapter 5, "Implementing Systematic Test Development," which explains the development of test blueprints, elaborates on how intermediate-level general objectives can be applied across course content, and how they guide the development of a test blueprint to establish content-related evidence of test validity.

Number of Learning Outcomes

How many learning outcomes should you identify for each objective? Obviously there is no standard answer to this question. Linn and Gronlund point out that it is impossible to identify every possible behavior that is associated with a developmental-level objective. They suggest that there is no advantage to listing more than seven or eight outcomes for each objective. The important thing is to make the list as representative as possible, so it reflects the behaviors that demonstrate the achievement of the objective (2000, p. 67).

Utilizing Instructional Objectives

Once objectives and outcomes are established, it is important to share them with students and to use them as a guide for course development. Reilly and Oermann (1990, p. 48) identify the following three directions provided by instructional objectives:

1. The teaching activity best suited to meet the objective

2. The type of learning activity which enables the learner to accomplish the behavior desired in the outcome

3. Methods and criteria for evaluation of the attainment of the objective.

Instructional objectives provide a road map for selecting teaching approaches, creating learning activities, and determining the methods for assessing outcomes. Examine the objective presented in Figure 3.4. Note that it designates learning outcomes in all three learning domains—cognitive, affective, and psychomotor. Therefore, a variety of teaching/learning and assessment strategies are required in order to address this objective. The psychomotor component certainly suggests that the teaching activities include a demonstration of the activity; while the cognitive and affective components suggest activities that might include lecture, computer-assisted instruction, and/or readings. An assortment of learning activities such as clinical or laboratory practice, process recordings, role playing, and written assignments should be incorporated into the plan to address each of the domains. Finally, assessment procedures should also include a variety of approaches, including written assignments, multiple-choice exams, laboratory observation, and clinical evaluation. With this design, the behaviors specified as desired outcomes direct all aspects of an educational experience.

Table 3.3 illustrates how teaching, learning, and assessment strategies can be planned to address all of the learning outcomes associated with an objective. Table 3.3 also demonstrates how strategies can overlap. A particular strategy can address multiple outcomes during the same experience, and strategies can be applied concurrently to different areas of the instructional process. Consider *written assignments*. This strategy can simultaneously be a learning activity and an assessment procedure, while it addresses several outcomes. The important point is that activities are planned to address every outcome in every area of the instructional process—teaching, learning, and assessment.

Criteria for Effective Objectives

Linn and Gronlund proposed a list of criteria to guide teachers in the development of instructional objectives. The list of criteria includes completeness, appropriateness, soundness, and feasibility (2000, p. 62). Effective objectives are also relevant, open-ended, written in terms of student behavior, and shared with students.

Complete

An objective should be included for each important aspect of a course. Knowledge objectives are easiest to include. Special attention must be paid to include objectives that focus on higher-order thinking skills as well as on the affective domain (Linn & Gronlund, 2000).

Appropriate

In order for the objectives to be relevant, they must be congruent with the general goals of the school, and they should be consistent with the program's mission, goals,

TABLE 3.3 Worksheet for Instructional Strategies Based on Learning Outcomes

Objective: At the conclusion of instruction the student will safely perform basic nursing procedures

Learning Outcomes	Teaching Strategies			Learning Activities				Assessment Procedures				
	Readings	CAI	Demonstration	Lecture	Written Assignments	Role Playing	Journal	Clinical/Lab Practice	Multiple-Choice Exams	Journal	Clinical/Lab Observation	Written Assignments
Identify the rationale for the procedure.	X	X		X	X		X		X	X	X	X
Acknowledge the impact of the procedure on the client.	X	X		X	X	X	X				X	X
Describe the steps of the procedure.	X	X	X	X	X	X		X	X		X	X
Explain the procedure to the client.	X	X		X			X		X	X	X	
Select the appropriate equipment for the procedure.	X	X	X	X				X	X		X	X
Perform the procedure with a predetermined degree of accuracy.		X	X					X		X		X
Maintain appropriate aseptic technique during the procedure.	X	X	X	X				X		X		X
Interpret client responses to the procedure.	X	X		X			X	X	X	X		X
Communicate the results of the procedure appropriately.	X				X		X	X	X	X	X	X
Provide client follow-up based on the results of the procedure.	X	X		X			X		X		X	X

and outcomes (Linn & Gronlund, 2000). The majority of the objectives in a nursing program should address developmental-level learning and should also reflect the progress in the attainment of developmental learning.

Sound

Sound objectives are in harmony with the principles of teaching and learning. They must be appropriate to the educational and experience level of the students. Objectives that relate to the students' needs and build on prior experience will appropriately motivate students. Objectives should also reflect outcomes that are permanent. Students will retain knowledge that is meaningful to them. Objectives that are perceived as trivial will be dismissed by learners. The nature of the learning reflected in the objectives should be permanent. Learning assumes relevance for the students when the outcomes, which are applicable to a specific situation, are transferable to other real-world situations (Linn & Gronlund, 2000).

Feasible

Clearly defined and attainable objectives are more valuable than a long list of unattainable goals. Teachers should consider whether the objectives are realistic and attainable in terms of student ability, available time, and instructional resources. Unrealistic goals discourage both students and teachers and soon become meaningless (Linn & Gronlund, 2000).

Relevant

Relevant objectives can help decrease the trivia in an educational experience by focusing teachers on what is important in a course of instruction (Reilly & Oermann, 1990). Once appropriate objectives are identified, teachers are then compelled to identify teaching, learning, and assessment strategies that address the required outcomes of the objectives. A teacher must answer the following questions: "Why am I using this strategy? What purpose does it serve?"

Open-Ended

Objectives should be clear enough to define student behavior. They should provide direction without limiting the learning experience. An objective that prescribes strict methodology limits both students and teacher because it constrains the way students can demonstrate the behavior, and it requires the teacher to only assess student performance in terms of the specified method (Reilly & Oermann, 1990). Consider this example of a restricted objective:

Demonstrates safe nursing practice by accurately performing procedures.

This objective suggests that only an accurate performance of the procedures demonstrates safety. In addition, it ignores the other criteria specified by the learning outcomes in Figure 3.4 that operationalize safe performance of nursing procedures. Writing objectives that are restricted in this manner requires that you develop an extensive and cumbersome list of objectives in order to address all of the important aspects of a course.

Open-ended objectives provide you with more flexibility. When they are content-free, it is possible to add specific learning outcomes and use the same list of objectives across units of study (Linn & Gronlund, 2000, p. 65).

Delineate Student Behavior

Outcomes for each objective should identify the student behavior that defines and signifies achievement of the objective. When objectives are written with outcomes in terms of student behavior that describes learning, they clarify your instructional intent and provide the basis for teaching methods, learning activities, and assessment strategies.

Shared with Students

This may seem too obvious to even mention, but it is very important and it must be emphasized. If you follow the criteria to develop effective objectives (Figure 3.9), implement a plan to promote learning attainment, and develop assessments based on your objectives, the objectives will truly be meaningful and students will appreciate their value. There is no point to simply giving *lip service* to an instructional plan. When students believe that you mean what you say, and that your objectives truly reflect what is expected of them, they are provided with a framework for assessing their own progress and identifying their own strengths and weakness. In fact, they are encouraged to assume responsibility for their own learning. Sharing meaningful objectives with students encourages the pursuit of life-long learning by empowering them to develop their own plan for directing their activities toward meeting objectives.

Criteria for Effective Instructional Objectives

- Complete
- Appropriate
- Sound
- Feasible
- Relevant
- Open-ended
- Delineate Student Behaviors
- Shared with Students

FIGURE 3.9   The criteria for effective instructional objectives

Summary

Instructional objectives are the foundation for teaching, learning, and assessment in education. Not only are they the first step in establishing the validity of our instructional methods and assessments, they actually serve to expedite the process of systematic course development. The outcomes associated with these objectives are the common thread that is woven through all aspects of an instructional course. They provide the structure that helps educators to organize and communicate their instructional intent; they direct the development of teaching and learning strategies; and they form the basis for the development of measurement instruments. Because of the critical role they play, it is imperative that you invest the effort in developing clearly written instructional objectives and learning outcomes as the initial step in the development of an instructional course.

4 Assessing Critical Thinking

"Minds are like parachutes.
They only function when they are open."

—Sir James Dewar

In this age of increasing complexity and accelerating change, there is a growing acknowledgment that the focus of education at all levels must shift from the transmission of information to the development of critical thinking skills. Paul (1993) equates the self-disciplined, open-minded habits of critical thinking with the survivor skills needed in the real world of the 21st century. Paul maintains that in order to encourage the growth of individuals who will be able to cope with a complex society, educators must abandon the practice of teaching students what *to think, and instead focus on teaching them* how *to think.*

Teaching, learning, and assessment are interwoven in the instructional process. When this process involves the promotion of higher-order thinking, such as critical thinking, educators are presented with a unique set of challenges. The assessment principles presented in Chapters 2, "The Language of Assessment," and Chapter 3, "Developing Instructional Objectives," form the basis for developing valid and reliable measurement instruments. When you apply these principles of assessment to the complex construct of critical thinking, you must expand your thinking to define the construct and to identify the outcomes that form the basis for valid measurement instruments. As with all assessments, an assessment of critical thinking requires that you select the method that best suits the objective. Multiple-choice exams are one of the methods that can be used to effectively assess learning outcomes related to critical thinking.

Accreditation Outcomes

Today's health care arena is certainly one of the most complex environments in society. The vast body of nursing knowledge combined with continuous technological advances and the economic pressure on the health care system require that nurses have finely tuned, critical thinking skills (Jacobs, Ott, Sullivan, Ulrich, & Short, 1997). The ability to think critically, make decisions, and formulate independent judgments are skills that are essential for safe nursing practice in today's diverse and complex health care environment (Pond, Bradshaw, & Turner, 1991).

Thus, nurse educators are faced with the challenge of providing student nurses with a strong foundation in critical thinking. The NLNAC has formalized this challenge by designating critical thinking as one of the required educational outcomes for the accreditation of post-secondary and higher degree nursing programs (NLNAC, 2000). The NLNAC Standard VI: Educational Effectiveness (see Figure 4.1) requires that, "The program has an identified plan for systematic evaluation and assessment of educational outcomes" (p. 20). In order to satisfy this standard, nursing faculty must develop a written plan for systematic program evaluation for five required outcomes, as well as for two elective outcomes. As part of the systematic program evaluation, the NLNAC directs each program to define the constructs and identify assessment measures for each of the required and elective outcomes.

NLNAC
Standard VI: Educational Effectiveness

Required Outcomes:

- Critical thinking
- Communication ability
- Therapeutic nursing interventions
- Patterns and rate of employment
- Performance on NCLEX and certifying examinations

FIGURE 4.1   NLNAC required outcomes

Establishing Evidence of Validity

In the discussion related to establishing construct-related evidence of validity in Chapter 2, "The Language of Assessment," the need for a clear definition of the construct being measured is identified. Once a definition is established, objectives that correlate with the definition can be identified, and the learning outcomes that reflect the construct's characteristics can be written in terms of measurable student behavior. This process facilitates the development of instructional strategies and instruments to measure the construct.

Critical thinking poses a challenge for instruction and measurement because it is a complex construct with no standard definition. In fact, credible definitions of critical thinking are too numerous to count. Yet, while most definitions are distinctly individual in their emphasis and approach, they are often noticeably consistent with each other. Many definitions agree that critical thinking involves attitude, knowledge and skills (Ennis, 1985; Facione, Facione, & Sanchez, 1994; Ford & Profetto-McGrath, 1994; Kataoka-Yahiro & Saylor, 1994; Koch & Speers, 1997; Miller & Malcolm, 1990; Oermann & Gaberson, 1998; Paul, 1993).

Defining Critical Thinking in Nursing

Critical thinking definitions, which are applied to the practice of nursing, often focus on the need for critical thinking ability in decision making, problem solving, and clinical judgment (Adams, 1999; Bandman & Bandman, 1995; Case, 1994; Green, 2000; Jacobs, et al., 1997; Miller & Malcolm, 1990; Pardue, 1987; Videbeck, 1997). The nursing process is frequently identified by educators as the context in which critical thinking skills are applied (Conger & Mezza, 1996; Miller & Malcolm, 1990; O'Sullivan, Blevins-Stephens, Smith, & Vaughn-Wrobel, 1997). However, several authors identify that the nursing process is not an adequate conceptualization of critical thinking in the current health care environment (Kataoka-Yahiro & Saylor, 1994; Koch & Speers, 1997).

Critical thinking in nursing is frequently described as being discipline-specific; requiring a sound knowledge base (Ford & Profetto-McGrath, 1994; Kataoka-Yahiro & Saylor, 1994; White, Beardslee, Peters, & Supples, 1990). Ford and Profetto-McGrath reviewed the nursing literature in support of their observation that problem-solving is the prevailing conceptualization of critical thinking in nursing curricula. They assert that the problem-solving model maintains the status quo, and they propose a model of critical thinking in the curriculum as praxis, where critical reflection mediates between authentic knowledge and autonomous action.

In the NLNAC's *Planning for Ongoing Systematic Evaluation and Assessment of Outcomes,* critical thinking is defined as "the deliberative nonlinear process of collecting, interpreting, analyzing, drawing conclusions about, presenting, and evaluating information that is both factually and belief based. In nursing, this is demonstrated by clinical judgment which includes ethical, diagnostic and therapeutic dimensions; and research" (2000, p. 8).

Rubenfeld and Scheffer conducted a research study which used the Delphi method to identify the essence of critical thinking in nursing. An international panel of nurses participated in the study, and the following consensus statement was generated:

Critical thinking in nursing is an essential component of professional accountability and quality nursing care. Critical thinkers in nursing exhibit these habits of the mind: confidence, contextual perspective, creativity, flexibility, inquisitiveness, intellectual integrity, intuition, open-mindedness, perseverance, and reflection. Critical thinkers in nursing practice the cognitive skills of analyzing, applying standards, discriminating, information seeking, logical reasoning, predicting, and transforming knowledge (2000, p. 5).

From reports of research studies to descriptions of strategies promoting critical thinking in nursing, the nursing and education literature abounds with articles related to critical thinking. Yet, it must be clarified that there is not one universal definition of critical thinking in nursing. It is essential for each nursing program to delineate and take ownership of its own definition of critical thinking. Instructional objectives, learning outcomes, teaching-learning strategies, and measurement instruments evolve from a carefully constructed definition. The key to developing your own definition is to review the literature on critical thinking as a frame of reference for creating a definition of critical thinking that is congruent with your faculty's collective perspective of the construct.

Sample Definition of Critical Thinking in Nursing

In order to illustrate the principles of test construction, I have carefully examined numerous definitions of critical thinking and have developed a sample definition of critical thinking as it applies to nursing (refer to Figure 4.2).

Critical thinking in nursing is discipline-specific, reflective reasoning that guides the process of deciding what to do or believe in unique situations.

FIGURE 4.2   Definition of critical thinking

Note that although this definition describes critical thinking, it is a very general one and does not provide a clear direction for guidance in developing instructional strategies or measurement instruments to assess the construct. Consider the expanded definition shown in Figure 4.3. Including the characteristics of critical thinking in this expanded definition establishes the criteria that define the construct, and also provides a basis for developing instructional objectives.

Critical thinking in nursing is discipline-specific, reflective reasoning that guides the process of deciding what to do or believe in unique situations. The critical thinker possesses an analytical attitude, demonstrates sensitivity to context, questions assumptions, bases inquiry on credible sources, considers a variety of solutions, and pursues ongoing evaluation.

FIGURE 4.3   An expanded definition of critical thinking

Instructional Objectives and Learner Outcomes

Once you have defined a construct, you are ready to establish objectives that will guide you in planning instructional and assessment activities. The expanded definition of critical thinking easily translates to an instructional objective with learning outcomes. Figure 4.4 represents a general critical thinking instructional objective with the characteristics of critical thinking, as shown in Figure 4.3, identified as the learning outcomes.

At the conclusion of the course, the student will demonstrate skill in critical thinking in health care situations as evidenced by:

- Displaying an analytical attitude

- Demonstrating sensitivity to context

- Questioning assumptions

- Basing inquiry on credible sources

- Considering a variety of solutions

- Pursuing ongoing evaluation

FIGURE 4.4   Critical thinking instructional objective with characteristics as learning outcomes

The learning outcomes specified in the instructional objective are the characteristics that are specified in the definition. Although the learning outcomes are measurable, note that they are not nearly as specific as the outcomes identified in Figure 3.4 in Chapter 3, "Developing Instructional Objectives." The explanation is obvious: Figure 3.4 represents a mastery level instructional objective that has a limited behavior domain with a sequential learning process. Behaviors, which define the objectives at a mastery level, are readily identified.

In contrast to mastery-level learning, critical thinking represents higher-order, developmental-level learning; it is a complex construct that is not easily defined. The domain of this construct is limitless, and its learning does not proceed in a sequential manner. Critical thinking skills are not easily obtained. In fact, many argue that becoming a critical thinker involves a life-long process of learning. Because of their developmental nature, instructional objectives for critical thinking should focus on a continuous development of skills.

In order to further clarify the meaning of an objective for a complex construct, a third level can be added to the objective (see Figure 4.5). This level identifies a sample of behaviors that demonstrate the achievement of the learning outcomes (Linn & Gronlund, 2000). However, before we can develop this third level, we must first identify the measurable behaviors that define each characteristic of the construct.

Tri-Level Instructional Objective

Level I: Construct (Objective)

Level II: Characteristic of construct (Learning Outcome)

Level III: Indicators of achievement of the learning outcome (Specific Behaviors)

FIGURE 4.5   Template for a tri-level instructional objective

Critical thinking is an example of a construct for which behaviors can be identified to denote progress in attaining the characteristics that define the construct. These behaviors are the specific tasks that represent how students exhibit achievement of each learning outcome, which in turn provides evidence of progress toward achieving the objective. The third level provides relevant measures, which demonstrate the achievement of the learning outcomes that are characteristic of the construct of higher-order thinking, such as critical thinking. Using this model, the construct then forms the objective, the characteristics form the learning outcomes, and the specific behaviors provide the indicators of achievement of the learning outcomes.

Behaviors Associated with the Characteristics of Critical Thinking

What behaviors demonstrate the identified learning outcomes of critical thinking? For example, what evidence will you accept to validate that a student *maintains sensitivity to context*? By identifying the specific behaviors that define the characteristics, you set the stage for the creation of learning strategies and measurement instruments, and also provide students with a clear understanding of your expectations.

How can behaviors be linked to the characteristics that are identified in a definition of critical thinking? By carefully analyzing the characteristics that define critical thinking, you can identify measurable behaviors that provide evidence of the characteristics. The lists of observable behaviors that follow may seem long. However, it is wise to identify a comprehensive list for each characteristic. You will then have a broad selection of defining behaviors to choose from later on when you write your instructional objectives.

Possesses an Analytical Attitude

A critical thinker has the disposition to think critically and is willing to be open minded and question the assumptions that underlie the customary ways of thinking. A critical thinker recognizes that it is far easier to be passionate in defense of what one believes than to comprehend why somebody believes something different.

In fact, one can have the ability to think critically, but be unwilling to do so. An egocentric, dogmatic attitude will prohibit an individual from becoming a critical thinker, even if this individual intellectually understands the concepts associated with critical thinking. An analytical attitude motivates an examination of assumptions, which are the basis for how we think and act. Behaviors that evidence this quality include, but are not limited to

- Has a steadfast commitment to inquiry

- Is confident of own abilities

- Pursues facts rather than defends beliefs

- Accepts challenges to own beliefs

- Is willing to relinquish own beliefs

- Maintains an impartial and open-minded approach

- Seeks out a variety of viewpoints

- Considers the feelings and beliefs of others

- Changes viewpoint when the situation warrants it

- Engages in dialogical thinking

- Reflects on own thinking

- Practices metacognition

- Maintains flexibility

- Upholds intellectual integrity

- Is proactive rather than reactive

Demonstrates Sensitivity to Context

A critical thinker is a practical problem-solver who recognizes that each situation is unique and explores issues in context. Behaviors that evidence this quality include, but are not limited to

- Identifies actual and potential health care problems, concerns, and issues

- Reframes problems, concerns, and issues in context

- Seeks to understand the client as a unique person

- Formulates a strategy to obtain needed information

- Asks relevant questions

- Solicits client's perspective

- Examines subjective and objective data

- Clarifies the meaning of information

- Collects data from all relevant sources

- Decodes the significance of the data

- Organizes data in a systematic manner

- Identifies the need for additional data

- Establishes plan for the individual situation

- Identifies worth of plan to client

Questions Assumptions

A critical thinker maintains a healthy skepticism when analyzing data. A critical thinker looks for assumptions behind thinking and is open to alternative ways of viewing the world. Behaviors that evidence this quality include, but are not limited to

- Examines presumptions about how the world works

- Seeks alternative viewpoints

- Recognizes that there is more than one normal pattern

- Clarifies beliefs and value judgments

- Looks for evidence behind beliefs

- Separates facts from fallacy

- Distinguishes fact from opinion
- Identifies faulty reasoning
- Compares and contrasts ideas and beliefs
- Investigates unsubstantiated claims
- Validates assumptions underlying conclusions

Bases Inquiry on Credible Sources

A critical thinker uses a systematic, sequential thinking process to discriminate between accurate and inaccurate evidence. Your capacity for critical thinking increases as your knowledge base increases. Behaviors that evidence this quality include, but are not limited to

- Uses a systematic, sequential thinking process
- Organizes information
- Operates from a sound, domain-specific knowledge base
- Recognizes limitations of own knowledge
- Utilizes valid reference resources
- Identifies when a problem, issue, or concern exists
- Suspends judgment while focusing on what to believe
- Analyzes data based on knowledge base
- Validates data based on knowledge base
- Recognizes assumptions
- Identifies limitations of data
- Weighs evidence for accuracy and relevance
- Discriminates between accurate and inaccurate evidence
- Distinguishes between relevant and irrelevant information
- Selects pertinent information
- Considers professional, ethical, and legal standards
- Makes inferences based on data

Considers a Variety of Solutions

A critical thinker collaborates with clients and other health care providers to consider a variety of alternatives when selecting and implementing solutions. Behaviors that evidence this quality include, but are not limited to

- Guides collaborative process
- Poses creative solutions to unique problems

- Examines alternative solutions

- Evaluates the integrity of conclusions

- Respects the knowledge level of others

- Develops a plan of action

- Provides a scientific rationale for plan

- Prioritizes interventions

- Predicts outcomes

Pursues Ongoing Evaluation

A critical thinker habitually seeks new information and identifies new evidence to serve as the basis for future inquiries. Behaviors that evidence this quality include, but are not limited to

- Evaluates the effect of a plan from a variety of perspectives, including the client, family, and other health care providers

- Seeks objective information to validate effectiveness of the plan

- Analyzes new information

- Obtains input and criticism from others

- Draws conclusions about the plan's effectiveness

- Develops the criteria for evaluation

- Revises a plan when the evidence warrants

Tri-Level Critical Thinking Objective

Adding a third level to an objective for a complex construct helps clarify the learning outcomes for both student and teacher. Remember that it is impossible to identify the universe of behaviors that describe developmental learning. The behaviors previously identified for each of the characteristics of critical thinking, provide long, although not comprehensive lists. Yet, even these lists are too cumbersome to be included in their entirety when specifying learning outcomes for classroom instruction. In the end, it is your professional judgment that makes the final decision. Start by developing a comprehensive list of specific behaviors and then select a sample from that list of behaviors that indicate achievement of the outcome in your course.

It is important to identify a sample of defining behaviors for each characteristic before you decide what assessment techniques to use. The outcomes should guide the teaching and learning strategies and assessment procedures, the strategies and procedures should not determine the outcomes. Identify the outcomes and behaviors first, and then let them guide the development of the instructional process.

Table 4.1 illustrates the levels that define a tri-level critical thinking instructional objective. In this example, the construct forms the objective, the characteristics form the learning outcomes, and the selection of specific behaviors provides evidence of achievement of the learning outcomes.

TABLE 4.1   Three Levels for a Critical Thinking Instructional Objective

(Level I)   Demonstrates skill in critical thinking in health care situations by

(Level II)   Demonstrating sensitivity to context.

(Level III)

- Asks relevant questions.

- Solicits the client's perspective.

- Identifies situations requiring modification.

- Establishes priorities for the individual situation.

- Verifies the value of the plan to the client.

The tri-level critical thinking objective in Table 4.1 addresses one characteristic or learning outcome of critical thinking—"*Demonstrating sensitivity to context.*" Level III of the objective specifies five specific observable behaviors selected by the teacher that provide evidence that the student is demonstrating the characteristic. Note that these behaviors were chosen from the long list of behaviors that were previously identified as defining the characteristic of "demonstrating sensitivity to context." There is no formula for selecting the specific behaviors. It is your professional judgment that determines which behaviors are relevant for your instructional course.

It is important to note that the specific observable behaviors are not learning outcomes in their own right; they are simply behaviors that are acceptable as indicators of achievement of the learning outcome (Linn & Gronlund, 2000, p. 69). For example, the behaviors of the third level in Table 4.1—asks, solicits, identifies, establishes, and verifies—represent specific actions that indicate the ability to "*demonstrate sensitivity to context.* Your goal is not to teach students how to ask or identify. Students should be able to demonstrate sensitivity to context. Thus, the specific behaviors represent how students exhibit the achievement of the learning outcome. The third level of specific responses provides a transition between the learning outcomes and the relevant measures that assess the construct of higher-order thinking.

Table 4.2 presents a complete tri-level instructional objective for critical thinking. Each of the six characteristics is included as a learning outcome. Note that the behaviors identified in the third level are all selected from the lists of behaviors previously identified for defining each characteristic.

Critical Thinking Assessment Plan

The complex nature of the critical thinking construct requires that complex measures are employed when implementing both instructional approaches and assessment techniques. Certainly the didactic approach that is common in classroom instruction must be replaced by more innovative techniques that teach our students *how* to think, rather than *what* to think. Exploring the behaviors, which characterize critical thinking, and the learning outcomes, which operationalize the construct, will help you to identify the approaches you can use to foster critical thinking in your students.

TABLE 4.2   A Comprehensive Critical Thinking Tri-Level Instructional Objective

Demonstrates skill in critical thinking in health care situations by

1. Displaying an analytical attitude
   1.1 Pursues facts
   1.2 Seeks a variety of viewpoints
   1.3 Practices metacognition
   1.4 Maintains flexibility
   1.5 Is proactive rather than reactive

2. Demonstrating sensitivity to context
   2.1 Asks relevant questions
   2.2 Solicits the client's perspective
   2.3 Identifies situations requiring modification
   2.4 Establishes priorities for the individual situation
   2.5 Verifies the value of the plan to the client

3. Questioning assumptions
   3.1 Examines presumptions about how the world works
   3.2 Seeks alternative viewpoints
   3.3 Separates fact from fallacy
   3.4 Compares and contrasts ideas and beliefs
   3.5 Validates the assumptions behind conclusions

4. Basing inquiry on credible sources
   4.1 Operates on a sound, domain-specific knowledge base
   4.2 Recognizes limitations of own knowledge
   4.3 Utilizes valid information sources
   4.4 Discriminates between accurate and inaccurate information
   4.5 Makes inferences based on data

5. Considering a variety of solutions
   5.1 Guides collaborative problem-solving process
   5.2 Examines alternative solutions
   5.3 Develops a plan
   5.4 Provides scientific rational for the plan
   5.5 Prioritizes interventions
   5.6 Predicts outcomes

6. Pursuing ongoing evaluation
   6.1 Evaluates the effect of the plan from a variety of perspectives, including those of the client, significant others, and other health care providers
   6.2 Seeks objective information to validate the effectiveness of the plan
   6.3 Analyzes new information
   6.4 Draws conclusions about the plan's effectiveness
   6.5 Develops criteria for evaluation
   6.6 Revises the plan when the evidence warrants

Once you have established your objectives, it is time to ask: "What learning activities will effectively promote the attainment of the outcomes I have established?" For example, what strategies can you implement to provide your students with the opportunity to *display an analytical attitude* or to *demonstrate sensitivity to context*? Clearly established objectives provide direction for both you and your students. A variety of valuable resources are available that propose creative teaching and learning strategies to promote critical thinking (for example, Alfaro-LeFevre, 1995; Angelo & Cross, 1993; Dexter, Applegate, Backer, Claytor, Keffer, Norton, & Ross, 1997; Diestler, 1998; Feingold & Perlich, 1999; Green, 2000; Jenkins & Turick-Gibson, 1999; Mastrian & McGonigle, 1999; Rubenfeld & Scheffer, 1999; Smith-Stoner, 1999; Weis & Guyton-Simmons, 1998).

Assessment of critical thinking poses issues that are as complex as the instructional challenges. In fact, instruction and assessment of this construct go hand-in-hand. Each characteristic must be carefully evaluated to identify the method that is most appropriate for assessment. In most cases, a multifaceted approach is necessary to fairly and accurately assess the behaviors associated with critical thinking. Instruments such as clinical evaluation tools, clinical and classroom discussions, portfolio assessments, case study analyses, projects, essays, and multiple-choice classroom exams are all appropriate mechanisms for the assessment of critical thinking. The foremost requirements are to match each learning outcome to the appropriate measurement instruments, and to gather as much information as you possibly can.

Multiple-Choice Exams and Critical Thinking

As discussed in the introduction, one premise of this book is that multiple-choice exams can contribute effectively to a multifaceted assessment of higher-order thinking. If you examine the previously defined behaviors associated with the characteristics of critical thinking, you will see that many of them are amenable to the development of multiple-choice items (see Table 4.3).

While this list illustrates that the behaviors associated with critical thinking can be measured with multiple-choice questions, it is by no means an exhaustive list. Remember, the domain of behaviors associated with critical thinking is virtually limitless. Therefore, it is very important for you to identify a sample of behaviors that represent progress toward the ultimate goal of becoming a critical thinker when developing your instructional objectives.

Note that some of the behaviors that were previously identified as defining the characteristics of critical thinking are not on the list in Table 4.3. Certainly, the most difficult attributes to measure with a multiple-choice exam are those relating to the affective domain. Because nurse educators have great opportunities to assess student achievement in the affective domain in both clinical and classroom environments, I would not include the characteristic *possesses an analytical attitude* in a blueprint for a multiple-choice classroom exam. I would instead focus on assessing that characteristic in a more qualitative manner.

TABLE 4.3　Critical Thinking Behaviors That Are Amenable to Multiple-Choice Items

Critical thinking multiple-choice items can be developed to assess the ability to

Demonstrate Sensitivity to Context
- Identifies situations requiring modification
- Asks relevant questions
- Distinguishes subjective from objective data
- Clarifies the meaning of information
- Collects data from relevant sources
- Decodes the significance of data
- Identifies the need for additional data
- Establishes priorities for the individual situation
- Delegates responsibility appropriately
- Recognizes safe practice

Question Assumptions
- Examines presumptions about how the world works
- Recognizes that there is more than one normal pattern
- Clarifies beliefs and value judgments
- Separates fact from fallacy
- Distinguishes fact from opinion
- Identifies faulty reasoning

Base Inquiry on Credible Sources
- Analyzes data based on accurate knowledge base
- Interprets data based on accurate knowledge base
- Recognizes assumptions and faulty reasoning
- Identifies the limitations of data
- Evaluates evidence for accuracy and relevance
- Discriminates between accurate and inaccurate evidence
- Distinguishes between relevant and irrelevant information
- Uses appropriate resources
- Incorporates professional, ethical, and legal standards
- Makes inferences based on data
- Bases actions on accurate information

Consider a Variety of Solutions
- Guides collaborative process
- Poses solutions to unique problems
- Examines alternative solutions
- Evaluates the integrity of conclusions
- Develops a plan of action
- Prioritizes nursing interventions
- Identifies a client's perception of plan
- Provides a scientific rationale for plan
- Establishes outcomes

Pursue Ongoing Evaluation
- Evaluates a plan's effect from a variety of perspectives
- Seeks objective information to evaluate the plan
- Analyzes new information
- Obtains input and criticism from others
- Draws conclusions about the plan's effectiveness
- Develops criteria for evaluation
- Revises a plan based on evaluation

Behaviors associated with other critical thinking characteristics are also omitted from the list in Table 4.3. Behaviors, such as *suspends judgment while focusing on what to believe*, which was previously cited as providing evidence for the characteristic, "bases inquiry on credible sources," are perhaps better assessed on an interpersonal level in a clinical setting. The behaviors that define the characteristics of critical thinking can be integrated through your assessment instruments and, as such, form the basis for the development of a systematic clinical and classroom critical thinking assessment strategy.

Table 4.4 illustrates how all of the identified characteristics of critical thinking can be evaluated with an integrated assessment plan. Once you decide which instruments are most suited to each characteristic, learning strategies and measurement instruments can then be tailored to meet the outcomes.

TABLE 4.4   Critical thinking assessment plan

Demonstrates Skill in Critical Thinking in Health Care Situations	Clinical Evaluation	Classroom MC Exams	Classroom Essay Exams	Case Study	Class Presentation	Journal
Possesses an Analytical Attitude	x					x
Demonstrates Sensitivity to Context	x	x	x	x	x	
Questions Assumptions	x	x	x	x	x	x
Uses Credible Sources	x	x	x	x	x	
Considers Various Solutions	x	x	x	x	x	
Pursues Ongoing Evaluation	x	x	x	x		x

Summary

Critical thinking skills are essential to the practice of nursing. The development of strategies to promote and assess these skills presents a challenge to nursing faculty. A clearly developed program definition is the first step in establishing construct-related evidence of validity for your classroom assessments. Identifying the characteristics of critical thinking and the behaviors that represent the characteristics, will guide your classroom instructional strategies and will also help you to identify quality standardized exams that meet your needs for assessing critical thinking.

Critical thinking is most effectively assessed though a systematically developed, multifaceted, integrated plan. Multiple-choice exams can play a valuable role in that plan. Chapter 5, "Implementing Systematic Test Development," presents guidelines for developing multiple-choice tests that include critical thinking outcomes. Chapter 6, "Developing Multiple-Choice Items," then addresses the techniques for developing multiple-choice items in detail, and Chapter 7, "Writing Critical Thinking Multiple-Choice Items," specifically identifies strategies for developing multiple-choice items that assess critical thinking.

5 Implementing Systematic Test Development

*"If you're not sure where you're going,
you're liable to end up someplace else—
and not even know it."*

—Robert Mager

Would you teach a course without developing a syllabus? Would you initiate a research project without a design? Would you compose a journal article without an outline? Most of you would answer with a resounding "No" to all of these questions. Yet, how many of you have approached test construction without a detailed plan?

When a teacher gives little thought to test preparation until the last minute, the results reflect the lack of effort. Grammatical and spelling errors, ambiguous questions, and clerical mistakes contribute to lack of face validity, which frustrates students. More importantly, the lack of planning results in tests that have poor reliability and fail to reflect the content and objectives of a course.

Initiating Test Development

A good test acknowledges the *informed* students and identifies those who are *uninformed* about course content and objectives. Effective measurement depends on careful planning. When you develop a test you must be concerned about the validity of the inferences you make based on the scores of the test. Content-related evidence of validity refers to the degree to which the test represents the course content, or how well the test represents the domain that is being tested. Unfortunately, evidence of content-related validity of teacher-made classroom measurements is frequently diminished by errors associated with the sampling of the course content and objectives. The key to assuring that the inferences you make based on your classroom tests are valid measures of student achievement lies in careful planning.

Test development refers to the process of producing a measurement by developing items and combining them to form a test according to a specified plan (AERA, et al., 1999, p. 37). In order to ensure that a test has representative content and objective sampling, development of a specified test plan should be part of course planning. Integrating test development into course planning establishes a foundation for evidence of validity.

In many nursing programs, several faculty members share the responsibility for teaching a course. When course responsibility is shared, it is imperative that one person be appointed to coordinate the activities of the course so that tests are produced in a timely manner. While the test coordinator has the ultimate responsibility for keeping the entire faculty group on track, all decisions related to the test should be made by consensus of the group.

Scheduling a Semester's Exams

Schoolcraft (1989) recommends developing a master plan based on your academic calendar for all of a course's exams before generating any individual test plans. An efficient method for initiating test development is to base the master plan on the content to be addressed in the course; the course's objectives can be incorporated later in the blueprinting process. When designing an overall plan for a semester's tests, it is important to schedule the tests so that the amount of content covered is proportional to the weight of the test in the final grade. Exams should be given frequently enough to allow for an adequate sampling of the content, and they should be spaced at reasonable intervals so students are not overwhelmed and have adequate time for learning.

Always consider school events when scheduling exams. The results of a test the day after a school dance, for example, may lead to invalid inferences. Flexibility that allows appropriate postponements can enhance the reliability and validity of your tests. As with each step of test development, using a systematic plan that incorporates your professional judgment expedites the process. Table 5.1 represents a sample master plan for a semester's exams.

Identifying the Purpose of the Test

Before you begin test development, you must decide what the purpose of the test is. Classroom tests can be used for a variety of purposes. Standard 1.2 of the *Standards for Educational and Psychological Testing* reminds us of the maxim that "no test is valid for all purposes." It requires that test developers clearly describe how test scores will be interpreted and used (AERA, et al., 1999, p. 17).

The items used on a test depend on the type of test you want to administer. If you are interested in determining the extent to which students have already achieved the objectives, you can administer a *pretest*. The goal of pretesting is to help a teacher identify the information to focus on during instruction and to assist students in identifying what they need to review. Items on a pretest are designed to determine what skills the students have already mastered.

TABLE 5.1   An Example of a Master Test Plan

Date	Exam	Content Area	Items	Final Grade Weight
10/12	Exam I			
		Unit I		
		Unit II		
			50	25%
11/20	Exam II			
		Unit III		
		Unit IV		
			50	25%
12/13	Comprehensive Final Exam			
		Unit I		
		Unit II		
		Unit III		
		Unit IV		
		Unit V		
		Unit VI		
		Unit VII		
			100	50%

The purpose of a *formative* test is to assess students during instruction. Questions for a formative test are directed at monitoring student progress, detecting problems, and providing feedback to both the student and the teacher. These tests usually cover a limited number of objectives and sample of course content (Linn & Gronlund, 2000).

Formative evaluation is more concerned with evaluating the teaching and developing appropriate instructional approaches than with assessing individual students (Trice, 2000). Therefore, it is usually not designed for the assignment of grades. If you use formative quizzes as graded assessments, be sure that students understand the grading implications. In any event, scores on formative quizzes should have less weight in the determination of the final course grade than summative evaluations.

Summative evaluation involves the process of assessing students in terms of the instructional objectives. Summative tests are designed to provide information about individual student achievement. A summative measurement presents questions that provide a representative sample of the objectives and content of a course. Summative tests are usually given at the end of a unit of study (unit exam) or at the end of a course (final exam) in order to assign a grade.

When a test is being administered to assign a grade, it is important to decide whether the test will be norm- or criterion-referenced. As Chapter 3, "Developing Instructional Objectives," discusses, when developmental-level learning is being measured it is beneficial to design criterion-referenced tests that are subject to norm-referenced interpretation. Furthermore, it is crucial that you clearly communicate the intent of a test to the students, so that they are aware of the implications of their test scores.

Determining the Length of the Test

How many questions will be on the test? Several elements enter into this decision. Those factors include the purpose of the measurement and the type of test items used. However, most often the main determinant is the amount of time allotted for the test. If one hour is allowed for an exam schedule, then you have to balance the blueprint so it covers the desired content and objectives over a reasonable number of items for that time period. A general rule of thumb for well-constructed, multiple-choice questions is to allow 60 minutes for every 50 questions. Chapter 6, "Developing Multiple-Choice Items," provides guidelines for developing clearly stated multiple-choice items that are presented in a format which students can read, understand, and answer in a one-minute time frame.

As you recall, speed can influence reliability. Speed should not be a factor in a test, unless the objective being measured relates to speed. Testing situations are anxiety-provoking in themselves. By adding severe time constraints, student anxiety will increase and interfere with performance. An essential requirement is to allow ample time for all of the students to complete all of the questions.

In many nursing programs, unit exams are limited to one hour and final exams are often administered in a two-hour period. If limits such as these dictate the number of questions that you can include on a test, you will need to schedule several exams during the semester. It is important to present the students with a sufficient number of test questions over the course of a semester so that you adequately sample the content and objectives of your course.

The practical issues associated with timing a test also are a reminder of the need to use a variety of assessment techniques. Assessment should not be confined to class time. Providing a variety of out-of-class assignments such as care plans, journals, and portfolio assessments increases the amount of information on which you can base your decisions. In addition, it also enables you to make informal (or formal, if you are so inclined and have the resources) correlations of your assessment measures. Remember the principle: The more assessment information you have, the more confidence you can have in your decisions.

Selecting What to Test

"The process of test development commonly begins with a statement of the purpose(s) of the test and the construct or content domain to be measured" (AERA, et al., 1999,

p. 37). The content and objectives measured by a test should be a representative sample of what was included in the course during the period covered by the test. The challenge of matching what is taught to what is assessed and how it is assessed requires careful planning and professional judgment. A blueprint is such a mechanism: It links the course content and objectives through the questions on a test.

Clear descriptions of *what* is to be assessed and *how* it is to be assessed are the first steps in test development. Ideally during course planning, the instructional objectives are identified, the content is mapped out, and exams are scheduled. The *what* of assessment is defined by the instructional objectives and the course content. The *how* is directed by the test plan, or blueprint. The objectives and course content serve as the framework for the blueprint.

Once the instructional objectives and course content are identified, the tests for the course can then be blueprinted. The tests can actually be prepared before instruction even begins. However, many teachers prefer to allow for unexpected course developments before finalizing an exam. Nevertheless, item development to meet a test plan should begin as soon as the blueprint is organized.

Selecting the Appropriate Assessment Format

Determining how well your students have achieved the instructional outcomes requires that you match each outcome with an appropriate assessment strategy. The more clearly you have stated your instructional objectives and learning outcomes, the more helpful they will be in assisting you in your decision on how to assess them. The challenge is to identify the most appropriate format for assessing the achievement of each instructional objective. The learning outcomes that are associated with the objectives provide the basis for determining how to assess the objectives.

The following basic types of measurement instruments provide a variety of formats that you can select:

1. *Selected-response* or supply-type items are also referred to as objective items because subjective judgment is not involved in scoring them. With these questions the correct answer is supplied and the student has to select it. Selected-response type items include the following:

   A. *True-false* items present a statement and the student must decide whether it is true or false. These items are easy to write and score. However, their use is limited to the testing of knowledge, and the potential for guessing is a concern.

   B. *Multiple-choice* items present a question or incomplete statement (stem) that is followed by two or more options. The student is required to select the correct or best choice to answer the question or complete the sentence. These items are easy to score, can test a broad content range, and lend themselves to objective analysis. Multiple-choice items can be written to assess higher-order thinking; however, well written items can be time-consuming to develop.

   C. *Matching* provides two lists of options and requires the student to select a choice from one list that parallels an option on the other list. These items are moderately easy to write and a broad range of content can be assessed. However, higher-order thinking is difficult to assess with this format.

2. *Constructed-response type items* are also referred to as subjective items because scoring can be open to interpretation. These items require the student to construct a response to a statement or question. These items include the following:

   A. *Completion* or *short answer* questions present the student with a question or a statement with one or more blanks. The student is required to provide a word, a phrase, or a sentence to complete the statement or to answer the question. These items are easy to write and can be administered in a short amount of time. However, verifying that the students have addressed the item criteria can make scoring time consuming.

   B. *Essay* questions ask a student to compose an original composition to respond to an idea or answer a question. These items can measure higher-order thinking skills and guessing is limited. Although the items are easy to write, scoring can be time consuming and only a limited content range can be assessed.

3. *Performance assessments* usually refer to assessments in which students are asked to perform. Usually there is no single right or wrong answer—a variety of responses can be considered excellent. There are numerous examples of performance assessment including oral presentations, experiments, journals, projects, case studies, and portfolio assessment. While performance assessments are particularly well suited for assessing higher-order thinking, they are subject to subjective interpretation and are time consuming to administer and score.

4. *Psychomotor assessment* is concerned with assessing motor skill performance. Psychomotor skills are essential in nursing practice because they are fundamental to safe practice. Motor skills also involve cognitive behavior, which directs the motor component, and results in a coordinated and productive performance (Reilly & Oermann, 1990). Psychomotor assessment involves observing a student's performance of motor skills and is also concerned with assessing the cognitive skills that are essential for the adaptation of procedures for safe nursing practice.

Each of these assessment formats has advantages and disadvantages. Your main concern is to select a method that is the most appropriate one for assessing a particular instructional objective. The specific behaviors that define the learning outcomes help guide the selection of the assessment format. When developing a multiple-choice exam, your first concern is to identify the objectives that can be assessed using this format. At the same time, it is critical to identify course objectives that cannot be assessed with a multiple-choice test and to develop a list of performance assessments to measure those outcomes.

Weighting the Content and Course Objectives

The worksheet shown in Table 5.2 represents the identification of objectives and content to be assessed by multiple-choice exams in a hypothetical course.

TABLE 5.2 A Content/Objectives Worksheet

A. Number of Unit Exams	2
B. Number of Items per Unit Exam	50
C. Total Unit Exam Items (A × B)	**100**
D. Number of Final Exam Items	100
E. Total Number of Exam Items (D + E)	**200**

Content	Lecture Hours	% of Hours	Number of Semester Items	OBJ 1 20%	OBJ 2 25%	OBJ 3 30%	OBJ 4 10%	OBJ 5 15%
Unit I	24	19%	36–40					
Unit II	20	16%	30–34					
Unit III	22	18%	34–38					
Unit IV	18	14%	26–30					
Unit V	14	11%	20–24					
Unit VI	14	11%	20–24					
Unit VII	14	11%	20–24					
Total	126 Hours		200 Items	38–42 Items	48–52 Items	58–62 Items	18–22 Items	28–32 Items

The content/objectives worksheet for semester exams in Table 5.2 is a form designed to assist you to systematically assign items for each content unit and course's objectives. Note that the form enables you to weight the content areas for an entire semester. The first step is to tally the total number of questions in all tests for a semester, and then identify the number of semester hours devoted to the course. Once the number of lecture hours for each content unit is identified, the percentage of the course that each content unit represents and the corresponding number of questions for each unit can be calculated.

In the hypothetical course presented in Table 5.2, there are 200 total semester exam items and 126 total semester lecture hours. By determining the percentage of the total lecture hours for each unit of content, it is easy to calculate the corresponding number of total exam items for each content area. For example, the 24 lecture hours for Unit One represents 19 percent of the 126 total lecture hours. Therefore, Unit One can be represented by 19 percent of the 200 total exam questions, or approximately 38 items. You will notice that a single value is not assigned to the number of items for each unit, rather a range is indicated For example, instead of 38 items for Unit One, the worksheet indicates a range of 36 to 40 items. This is far from an exact science—flexibility is important with test development.

The content is listed down the far left column on the worksheet, while the objectives are identified across the top row. Notice that the objectives are not equally weighted. Each objective is assigned a percentage. Assigning percentages to the objectives is a matter of professional judgment and it reflects the relative emphasis of the objective in the course. Note that percentage weight for each objective translates into a range of items, which can be included in assessing the objective on the exams over the semester. These ranges are indicated across the bottom row of the worksheet.

Determining the relative weight of a particular content area for a semester—based on the amount of class time devoted to that content—is a practical approach to blueprinting an exam. Although instructional time is not the only possible consideration for the weighting of content on a test, it is an important measure of the amount of emphasis given to each topic. It is only fair that the time devoted to the instruction of a particular content area should be a factor in determining its weight on a test. The percentage of instructional time devoted to each content area should correspond to the relative emphasis of each content area in the course, which then translates into the number of items for the content area on the exams.

While there are no hard and fast rules, the most effective approach for determining how many test items should deal with each unit of content in a semester's exams is to use a systematic procedure. Completing a content worksheet, such as the one shown in Table 5.3, systematizes the process of identifying items for specific content and simplifies the development of exam blueprints. This assignment should be a flexible one, with a range of items assigned to each content category.

The most significant criteria for establishing content-related evidence of validity is to have a representative sample of course content on your exams. To ensure this occurs, all units of content must be proportionately represented on exams over the course of the semester. Information from the content/objectives worksheet is used to complete a semester content item form. The worksheet in Table 5.3 maps out the distribution of content across the semester exams for the course represented in Table 5.2.

Note that in the course represented in Table 5.3, four of the content units are covered on unit exams and three are not. For example, Unit Two is allocated 16 percent of 200 items, or approximately 32 items for the entire semester. Because only Units One and Two are included in exam one, 21 to 25 of the 50 items on Exam One are from Unit Two. This number is arrived at because Unit Two represents 45 percent of the 44 lecture hours included on Exam One. Therefore, Unit Two can be apportioned an additional five to thirteen items for the final exam.

It is important to understand the purpose for taking the time to map out your exams in this highly specific manner. Units that are not tested during a semester should be more heavily represented on a comprehensive final exam than those units that were included on tests given during the semester. If they are not, there will not be valid representation of the course content on your exams. In order to fairly weight the blueprint, you need to identify how many items are devoted to each semester unit exam, so the areas that were not tested at all during the semester are adequately represented on the final exam.

Although the decisions made in apportioning items is somewhat arbitrary, you will find that the process ensures that your tests reflect the content emphasis of your course. The content worksheet in Table 5.3 will assist you in assigning items in proportion to the course content they represent, and will form the basis for establishing your test blueprints.

TABLE 5.3 Sample Content Item Worksheet

A. Number of Unit Exams	2
B. Number of Items per Unit Exam	50
C. Total Unit Exam Items (A × B)	**100**
D. Number of Final Exam Items	100
E. Total Number of Exam Items (D + E)	**200**

Total Lecture Hours	126	Total Exam Items	200				

Content Area	Lecture Hours	% of Total Lecture Hours	% of Exam Lecture Hours	Total Number of Items for Unit	Exam I Items	Exam II Items	Final Exam Items
Unit I	24	19%	55%	36–40	25–29		7–15
Unit II	20	16%	45%	30–34	21–25		5–13
Exam I					**50**		
Unit III	22	18%	55%	34–38		27–29	7–11
Unit IV	18	14%	45%	26–30		21–25	2–8
Exam II						**50**	
Unit V	14	11%		20–24			20–24
Unit VI	14	11%		20–24			20–24
Unit VII	14	11%		20–24			20–24
Total	**126 Hours**			**200 Items**	**50 Items**	**50 Items**	**100 Items**

Developing a Test Blueprint

Once you have completed a content worksheet, you are ready to prepare a test blueprint. A blueprint is a test plan that links the test items to the content and instructional objectives of the course, and provides a foundation for establishing content-related evidence of validity. Generating a blueprint before developing the test is essential for establishing evidence for the validity of the inferences made about the test scores.

A blueprint consists of a two-way chart that relates the instructional objectives to the course's content. It incorporates a list of objectives suitable for objective testing and a content worksheet that identifies the relative emphasis of what is included in the course. The chart ensures that the content and each of the learning outcomes receives appropriate emphasis on the test (Linn & Gronlund, 2000).

Table 5.4 represents a completed blueprint worksheet for the course represented in Tables 5.2 and 5.3. The instructional objectives, which the teacher has identified as being appropriate for assessment by multiple-choice test items, are listed across the top row and the units of content are listed down the first column of the chart. This is not a rigid process—flexibility is built in. Therefore, the items for each unit exam and the final exam are expressed as a range, and are transferred from the worksheet in Table 5.3 to their corresponding content units. The number of items for each objective is also expressed as the range identified in Table 5.2.

TABLE 5.4   Blueprint Worksheet

	Questions	OBJ 1 20%	OBJ 2 25%	OBJ 3 30%	OBJ 4 10%	OBJ 5 15%	Total
Range		38–42	48–52	58–62	18–22	28–32	200
Unit I	25–29	5	4	7	4	6	26
Unit II	21–25	5	8	8	1	2	24
Exam I	**50**	**10**	**12**	**15**	**5**	**8**	**50**
Unit III	27–29	7	10	1	2	7	27
Unit IV	21–25	4	4	10	3	2	23
Exam II	**50**	**11**	**14**	**11**	**5**	**9**	**50**
Unit I	10–14	5	2	3	0	2	12
Unit II	6–10	4	0	2	4	0	10
Unit III	7–11	4	1	0	0	2	7
Unit IV	3–7	0	0	3	3	0	6
Unit V	20–24	2	8	10	0	4	24
Unit VI	20–24	6	5	6	2	2	21
Unit VII	20–24	0	8	8	2	2	20
Final	**100**	**21**	**24**	**32**	**11**	**12**	**100**
Total	**200**	42	50	58	21	29	

Note that not all objectives are included in every content area on the blueprint worksheet in Table 5.4. Some of the cells on the chart are zero because every objective does not have to be assessed in every content area. The overall assessment of each of the objectives and content areas is in accordance with the specifications from Table 5.2.

The crucial concerns are that the assessment methods reflect the emphasis of course instruction (Linn & Gronlund, 2000) and that provisions are made to assess every objective and learning outcome.

Although the process of preparing a blueprint as detailed as the one illustrated in Table 5.4 may initially appear very time consuming, it actually promotes efficient test development. However, it is not essential that the blueprint be as detailed as the one presented. If you want to start slowly while you are learning this process, you may prefer to use the chart proposed in Table 5.2 and fill in a range of items in each of the cells. Be sure to be specific enough to ensure that your blueprints have enough detail to guide the development of meaningful, valid, and reliable test items—remember that the more detailed the blueprint is, the easier it is to write meaningful items.

Some teachers complete a detailed blueprint for the entire semester at a course's outset. Some teachers would rather identify the ranges for the content area and objectives, and then fill in the chart cells as the items are developed. Whichever approach you prefer, it is important that your blueprinting is done during course planning. As soon as the blueprint is prepared, item development and selection can be initiated.

The process of test development is becoming more streamlined with the advent of computer technology. Once you understand the techniques for blueprinting, your charts can easily be imported into a spreadsheet format. Electronic item banking programs are also available that include blueprinting in their test development process. In addition, once you have the capability of banking your items, item development is expedited. The benefits of implementing an item banking program are carefully examined in Chapter 12, "Instituting Item Banking and Test Development Software."

Reviewing the Blueprint

Once the blueprint is designed, it is essential that it is carefully examined to determine its relevance to the course. Professional test developers frequently use panels of recognized national experts to rate the relevancy of the blueprint to the domain being tested by an exam. Classroom teachers do not have this luxury. However, if you teach as part of a team, you can develop and review the blueprint as a group. Or, if you are the sole instructor, you can exchange blueprints and exams with a colleague for review.

The need for blueprint review introduces another reason for early preparation of tests. You cannot expect another faculty member to review your blueprint on a moment's notice. Nor is it realistic to expect members of a teaching team to be able to devote adequate time to carefully examining the relevancy of test items on short notice. The bottom line is the greater a time frame you allow for test development, the better the quality of your tests will be. A general rule of thumb is to have the blueprint ready for peer review during the planning phase of course preparation and to circulate each exam for final peer review three weeks before the scheduled exam date.

Blueprinting and item writing are the most time-consuming aspect of test development. Item banking software programs that develop blueprints, provide templates for word-processing, store items with data and references, have codes for classifying and querying, and enable easy access to thousands of items for test generation and revision based on data analysis are widely available. Even if you have limited computer expertise, these programs are user-friendly tools that can provide a useful mechanism for constructing and revising tests. Chapter 12, "Instituting Item Banking and Test Development Software," discusses these programs with suggestions for implementation in a nursing program.

The NCLEX-RN Test Plan

The test plan for the NCLEX-RN is a serious concern for nursing faculty. This examination reflects the knowledge, skills, and abilities that are the benchmarks for safe entry-level nursing practice (NCSBN, 2000). The 1998 test plan was developed from a 1996 job analysis study of newly licensed registered nurses (NCSBN, 1997). The job analysis is a nonexperimental, descriptive study that guides content distribution on the licensure exam and provides content-related evidence of validity (Yocum, 1999). The 1996 job analysis provided the framework for the 1998 NCLEX-RN test plan that directed the content included on the exam until April 2001.

Because changes occur in health care and nursing practice, job analysis studies are conducted every three years. Results of the most recent study, *Linking the NCLEX-RN National Licensure Examination to Practice: 1999 Practice Analysis of Newly Licensed Registered Nurses in the U. S.*, recommended that there be no substantial changes for the 2001 test plan (Hertz, Yocum, & Gawel, 1999). Therefore, the April 2001 test plan is essentially the same as the 1998 plan.

Four categories of client needs provide the framework for the current test plan. These categories are further divided into subcategories as follows (NCSBN, 2000, p. 4):

1. Safe Effective Care Environment
   A. Management of Care
   B. Safety and Infection Control

2. Health Promotion and Maintenance
   A. Growth and Development Through the Life Span
   B. Prevention and Early Detection of Disease

3. Psychosocial Integrity
   A. Coping and Adaptation
   B. Psychosocial Adaptation

4. Physiological Integrity
   A. Basic Care and Comfort
   B. Pharmacological and Parenteral Therapies
   C. Reduction of Risk Potential
   D. Physiological Adaptation

The test plan also addresses several processes that are fundamental to the practice of nursing. These concepts are not assigned percentages of representation in the test plan. Rather, they are integrated in a nonspecified manner, throughout the four categories of client needs. These integrated concepts and processes include (NCSBN, 2000, p. 4):

- Nursing Process
- Caring
- Communication and Documentation
- Cultural Awareness

- Self Care

- Teaching/Learning

Table 5.5 illustrates the percent range of the NCLEX-RN questions across the categories of client needs (NCSBN, 2000, p. 5).

TABLE 5.5   The NCLEX-RN Test Plan (effective date: April 2001)

A. Safe, Effective Care Environment	B. Health Promotion and Maintenance	C. Psychosocial Integrity	D. Physiological Integrity
1. Management of care (7–13%) 2. Safety and infection control (5–11%)	3. Growth and development through the life span (7–13%) 4. Prevention and early detection of disease (5–11%)	5. Coping and adaptation (5–11%) 6. Psychosocial adaptation (5–11%)	7. Basic care and comfort (7–13%) 8. Pharmacological and parenteral therapies (5–11%) 9. Reduction of risk potential (12–18%) 10. Physiological adaptation (12–18%)

Source: National Council of State Boards of Nursing. (2000) *Test plan for the national council licensure examination for registered nurses*. Chicago: Author.

You may notice that the NCLEX-RN test plan is not a two-way chart. That is because the current NCLEX-RN plan is a one-way classification system. The plan assigns a percentage of test questions only to the client needs categories and subcategories. Although they are integrated throughout the test, percentages for the integrated concepts are not specified.

Student success on the NCLEX-RN exam is a major concern for faculty. Issues such as accreditation, student recruitment, and even the very existence of a program are greatly impacted by student success or failure on this exam. Faculty are therefore understandably concerned with identifying strategies to promote student success. Because specific content is not included in the test plan, it is not possible to *teach to* this test, nor should that be the case. Following the guidelines for developing sound instructional strategies and the assessments that are presented in this book are the most effective methods for assisting students to be successful on the NCLEX-RN exam.

Table 5.6 provides a chart for an NCLEX-RN-based blueprint.

TABLE 5.6   An NCLEX-RN-Based Blueprint Chart

Content Area	A. Safe, Effective Care Environment		B. Health Promotion and Maintenance		C. Psychosocial Integrity		D. Physiological Integrity				Total
	1. Management of care (7–13%)	2. Safety and infection control (5–11%)	3. Growth and development through the life span (7–13%)	4. Prevention and early detection of disease (5–11%)	5. Coping and adaptation (5–11%)	6. Psychosocial adaptation (5–11%)	7. Basic care and comfort (7–13%)	8. Pharmacological and parenteral therapies (5–11%)	9. Reduction of risk potential (12–18%)	10. Physiological adaptation (12–18%)	
	1.	**2.**	**3.**	**4.**	**5.**	**6.**	**7.**	**8.**	**9.**	**10.**	**Total**
I.											
II.											
III.											
IV.											
V.											
VI.											
VII.											
VIII.											
IX.											
X.											
XI.											
XII.											

Total

Source: National Council of State Boards of Nursing. (2000). *Test plan for the national council licensure examination for registered nurses*. Chicago: Author.

This chart offers a column to include content that creates a two-way blueprint. It is counterproductive to blueprint your classroom exams using this method, because it is essential that you include your instructional objectives in your classroom blueprints. However, this chart can be useful for evaluating exams that purport to be NCLEX preparation tests. It is also useful as a cross-reference for evaluating your classroom exams.

Cross-Referencing Classroom Exams

Just as the NCLEX-RN test plan integrates several concepts and processes without specifically blueprinting them, you may also be interested in identifying constructs that are inherent in your exams, but not specifically represented on your blueprints. The nursing process in particular is an area of interest for most faculty. As Chapter 6, "Developing Multiple-Choice Items," addresses, nursing test questions are most effective when written in terms of the nursing process.

Tables 5.7, 5.8, and 5.9 provide cross reference grids for the nursing process, the cognitive levels, and client needs. While completing these grids will assist you with your test analysis, they can also be quite tedious to complete. However, as Chapter 12, "Instituting Item Banking and Test Development Software," discusses, item banking software enables you to easily code and classify items so that completing grids such as these is simply a matter of clicking your mouse.

TABLE 5.7   A Nursing Process Cross Reference Worksheet

	Exam I	Exam II	Exam III	Final
Assessment				
Analysis				
Plan/Implement				
Evaluate				
Total				

TABLE 5.8   A Cognitive Level Cross Reference Worksheet

	Exam I	Exam II	Exam III	Final
Knowledge/ Comprehension				
Analysis				
Application				
Total				

TABLE 5.9   Client Needs Cross Reference Worksheet

	A. Safe, Effective Care Environment 1. Management of care (7–13%) 2. Safety and infection control (5–11%)	B. Health Promotion and Maintenance 3. Growth and development through the life span (7–13%) 4. Prevention and early detection of disease (5–11%)	C. Psychosocial Integrity 5. Coping and adaptation (5–11%) 6. Psychosocial adaptation (5–11%)	D. Physiological Integrity 7. Basic care and comfort (7–13%) 8. Pharmacological and parenteral therapies (5–11%) 9. Reduction of risk potential (12–18%) 10. Physiological adaptation (12–18%)
Exam I				
Exam II				
Exam III				
Final				
Total				

Source: National Council of State Boards of Nursing. (2000) *Test plan for the national council licensure examination for registered nurses*. Chicago: Author.

Determining How Difficult a Test Should Be

There is no specific formula for deciding the difficulty level of a test. Items can be written at a wide range of difficulty levels; you can manipulate the complexity to make items more or less difficult. Your judgment is the best guide for determining the appropriate level of test difficulty.

The first consideration to make when deciding difficulty is the purpose of the test. Criterion-referenced tests do not consider the difficulty level of items, the only criterion is a student's attainment of a set of learning outcomes. Easy items are included in criterion-referenced tests, as long as they assess the learning outcome. Norm-referenced tests, on the other hand, are concerned with comparing student achievement. Norm-referenced tests aim to include items of average difficulty and to exclude items that are too easy. Finally, as Gronlund (1993) suggests, tests directed at assessing developmental-level learning should include items of varying difficulty.

Standardized tests often aim to have a mean of 0.50, with a difficulty range of approximately 0.3 to 0.8, to ensure a normal distribution of the scores. Items written within this range also provide the best discrimination indices. This approach would certainly yield a very difficult classroom test. Ideally, you should aim to have the average item difficulty equal to what you want the mean of the test to be. For example, if you are aiming for a test with a mean of 0.75, the average item difficulty should be 0.75. Because you are assessing developmental-level learning in nursing, you should include items at a higher difficulty level to identify those who are attaining higher achievement levels on the objectives. In doing so, you obtain a spread of scores on the test. In order to assess the behaviors that you expect all students to achieve, items that are easier than 0.75 difficulty must also be included on the test. These easier items are included to start the test off and to *offset* the harder items in order to achieve an average score of 0.75.

Identifying how difficult a new item will be is largely a matter of experience. Experienced teachers can often predict the approximate difficulty level of a test question. However, even experienced teachers can misjudge the way a question will work on a test. You must always be willing to examine the data analysis of a test and make adjustments based on that analysis. The test development software discussed in Chapter 12, "Instituting Item Banking and Test Development Software," offers teachers a great advantage for analyzing item and test data and for making adaptations to improve both the difficulty and discrimination levels of test items.

In addition, it is important to mention that the ability of the items to discriminate (i.e., distinguish between the high-achievers and the low-achievers on a test) is just as important as item difficulty. Chapter 6, "Developing Multiple-Choice Items," provides you with the extensive guidelines for item development that will improve the quality of your test questions. Chapter 10, "Interpreting Test Results," also provides information to help guide the improvement of the test items using item analysis data.

Preparing Students for a Test

Assessments should be designed to identify what students can do, not to minimize their performance. Classroom achievement tests should present opportunities for students to demonstrate their maximum ability. In order to perform at their peak, students need to be informed about what to expect, which includes the content and abilities that will be tested, what will be emphasized on the test, and how the test will be scored and weighted in the final grade (Nitko, 1996).

At the same time, you must be careful not to *teach to the test*. Addressing the content of specific questions gives students an unfair advantage and ruins the validity of your exams. Pretest content reviews present a particularly risky situation. Enthusiastic faculty members who want to see students succeed must be aware of the ethical implications of teaching to a test. While faculty are obligated to present students with fair assessments, they also have the same obligation to ensure that the students are meeting the course objectives. A test that has been shared with students, in any manner, is not a fair assessment.

"Pop Quizzes"

It is common practice to provide students with a syllabus at the outset of an instructional course. The syllabus usually includes the course objectives and content outline, the standards for grading, and the exam schedule. Providing a syllabus based on the belief that students should be informed about what to expect in the course promotes effective instruction.

Yet, many of the same teachers, who would never consider conducting a course without a syllabus, do not hesitate to surprise their students with unannounced quizzes. These *pop quizzes* were described by Nunnally in 1964 as "one of the few ways of hitting back at students now that corporal punishment is going out of fashion" (p. 105). Giving unannounced quizzes is the equivalent of not informing students.

Some may argue that these pop quizzes *keep students on their toes*. However, keeping students fully informed is a much better approach. How many teachers are precisely on schedule with every one of their assignments? How many nights have you been just too exhausted to correct another paper? How would you react if a supervisor *popped* in to evaluate you without notice? Sometimes, we seem to forget that students have lives too. Even the most conscientious student should be afforded the opportunity to plan course work in terms of a schedule. In order to plan, a student needs to know in advance what must be accomplished. Nitko recommends giving students at least 48 hours notice before any assessment (1996, p. 303).

Pop quizzes increase anxiety because they are associated with surprise. This anxiety is reduced when students can plan a study program. These assessments can also be patently unfair. Consider the student who is thoroughly prepared the week that there is no quiz, and who has a valid reason for being unprepared the week that there is one. Some students will even go through amazing logic exercises to figure out when quizzes will be given, and when the scheduled number are given, many students will feel that they are *off the hook*. These situations take the responsibility for learning away from the students. Teachers then become the *study police*, lying in wait to catch students who are not following the rules.

If you are concerned about providing incentives for students to keep up with course assignments, a good approach is to schedule a brief quiz on a set day each week. Give these quizzes minimal weighting in the final course grade, and allow students to drop one or two of their lowest grades. Thus, the anxiety of wondering whether a quiz will be given is removed, and the students are given responsibility for being prepared every week.

Sharing the Blueprint with Students

Should you give the test blueprint to students? While using a test blueprint can reduce student complaints that the test did not match the important content of the course (Tomey, 1999), there is a difference of opinion on whether to share the actual blueprint with the students. While students should be prepared for an upcoming assessment, some educators feel that sharing the blueprint *gives away* the test. This concern does not consider that the blueprint is simply a guideline. It does not specify test questions; it indicates the emphasis of the units of course content and the objectives on the test. Even if you were to list specific content topics on the blueprint, items written at the application and analysis levels require students to apply higher-order thinking to answer the questions correctly, and the outline thus would not be a *give-away* at all. A blueprint links the test items to the tasks required to demonstrate the mastery of a body of knowledge for the teacher, and it can serve this purpose for the students as well.

The most efficient way to share what is on a test is to share the test blueprint. Teachers share the objectives and content outline in the syllabus for every course. Sharing the test blueprints demonstrates to the students that the objectives really do matter and that teachers are not expecting rote memorization of the course content. Having a visual guide for how the objectives enter into the assessment equation makes their attainment more meaningful to students.

The blueprint shown in Table 5.4 is not necessarily suitable for sharing with students. Students need a moderate level of detail for a study guide. A chart similar to the one shown in Table 5.2 with a range of items included in each cell may be more appropriate. Whichever form you decide to use, it is important to share test blueprints with students to decrease their misconceptions, to help them to focus on the course objectives, and to provide them with the opportunity to demonstrate their maximum performance.

Table 5.10 summarizes the test development process.

TABLE 5.10 Guidelines for test development

A. Preliminary Considerations

1. Who will be the test coordinator?
2. How many tests are scheduled for the semester?
3. What is the purpose of the test?
4. How much time has been provided for the test?
5. How many items should be on the test?
6. What content will be covered by the test?
7. Will the test be criterion- or norm-referenced?
8. Which objectives are measured by the test?
9. What weight should be given to each of the content areas and objectives?
10. How difficult should the test be?
11. Which item formats are the most appropriate to use on the test?

B. Steps in Developing the Blueprint for an Objective Test

1. Determine the relative emphasis for the test.

   a. Decide the content weighting that accurately reflects the teaching emphasis.

   b. Identify the relative weight percentage for each objective.

2. Determine how many items should be written for each cell.

   a. Identify the range of items for each content area.

   b. Identify the range of items for each objective.

  c. Multiply the total number of items for a content area by the percentage assigned to the objective in each row.

  d. Use this figure as a guide to estimate a range of items for each cell on the blueprint worksheet.

3. Circulate the blueprint to faculty members for review.

C. Preparing the Test

1. Determine the faculty assignment based on number of items required for each cell.

2. Establish a due date for item submission.

3. Require the item writers to submit one item per page to the test coordinator.

4. The test coordinator edits and sorts the items according to the blueprint.

5. The test coordinator circulates the test items for review by the faculty members.

6. The test coordinator incorporates the suggestions made by the faculty for the items and assembles a final form of the test.

7. The test coordinator circulates the final form of the test for faculty edits.

8. Create a cover sheet, reproduce, number, and securely store the test until exam day.

Summary

Planning for classroom assessments is fundamental to establishing the validity of the inferences made based on test scores. Content-related validity refers to how closely a test represents the content domain of the course. The degree of content representativeness is a matter of fairness and is closely linked to careful planning. Determining a test's purpose and its content and objectives, how difficult the test should be, which item format to use, and how to weight the test's blueprint all need to be considered. If the purpose of an assessment experience is to enable students to demonstrate their maximum ability, then teachers must take every measure possible to maximize the fairness of that experience. This discussion also clarifies that developing blueprints for classroom exams provides an excellent source of content-related evidence of the validity of your exams.

6 Developing Multiple-Choice Items

"Good tests consist of good test items."

—Thomas Haladyna

While a good blueprint provides the foundation for a quality test, it does not guarantee quality results. The blueprint is only one step in the process. Careful attention must be focused on developing appropriate, well-crafted items that meet the specifications of the test plan. No matter how well developed the blueprint is, if the items fail to address the objectives and content of the course as specified in the blueprint, the validity of the test will be impaired. If ambiguously worded items are included on the test, students will be unable to decipher what is being asked, and the reliability of the test will be diminished. In either situation, inappropriate decisions could be made based on the test results.

Advantages of Multiple-Choice Items

The multiple-choice format is the most versatile type of test-item format. Those who object to multiple-choice items usually object to all objective test formats in favor of essay-type questions. While multiple-choice items do have limitations, they also have several advantages over essay-type questions.

When properly crafted, the multiple-choice format can be used to assess a wide range of learning outcomes across all cognitive levels. Multiple-choice items are adaptable to all types of subject matter; their scoring is accurate and efficient; and they provide students with practice for the types of items that they are likely to encounter on licensure and certification exams.

The issue of content sampling on a test is most efficiently addressed by the multiple-choice format. When compared to essay questions, multiple-choice items require much less time for recording answers. Therefore, multiple-choice exams can include many more items and afford a more representative sample of content on a test than constructed-response items, particularly essay questions.

While the constructed-response type format is susceptible to subjective scoring and poor test reliability, multiple-choice items provide objective measurement of student achievement and can be developed to yield higher test reliability. The difficulty level of multiple-choice items, which contributes to test reliability, is easier to control than with essay questions. Multiple-choice type items also lend themselves to item analysis, which enables the teacher to determine how well the items functioned with the group of students tested.

Multiple-choice items are compatible with efficient and accurate computerized scoring. In addition, item analysis data, which includes difficulty levels and discrimination indices of the items, can also be computer generated and used to improve the items. Last, but certainly not least, computer software can store multiple-choice items in an item bank for future use. Item banking, which is an invaluable tool for test development, is addressed in Chapter 12, "Instituting Item Banking and Test Development Software."

Limitations of Multiple-Choice Items

No item format or test is perfect. They all have flaws. Essay items are easier to construct than multiple-choice items, but they are time consuming to score and are susceptible to subjective scoring. On the other hand, multiple-choice items are time consuming to develop particularly because it is difficult to write the incorrect options. Multiple-choice items are easy to score, however, and they also lend themselves to the development of an item pool where items can be saved and improved based on item analysis for use on future tests.

Opponents of objective testing point out that the essay testing format is a more accurate measure of a student's ability to apply knowledge because it requires students to construct their own response, rather than to simply respond to a proposed answer. Another criticism of multiple-choice items is that they have a tendency to be written at the recall level. Even at higher cognitive levels, students might only need to recognize the correct answer; they do not need to organize and construct their own response. The format is also faulted because it is susceptible to guessing and tends to favor testwise students who can spot the clues in poorly written items.

Well-developed multiple-choice items can refute all of these criticisms. Effective multiple-choice items do not enable students to choose the correct answer by simple, rote memory. Rather, they require the student to reason out the basis for selecting the correct response. Carefully designed multiple-choice items eliminate the clues upon which testwise students depend. They can be designed so that students have to use critical thinking skills to make the subtle distinctions that are necessary to reason out the correct answer.

The debate over the qualities of different item formats should not be the main focus of test developers. One format is not inherently superior to another. Remember the basic principle: Select the item format that is most suitable for measuring the desired learning outcome. As Linn and Gronlund (2000) point out, while it is important to take advantage of the flexibility and applicability of the multiple-choice format, it should not be used when the objective requires performance-based assessment.

Multiple-choice items only fulfill their potential when they are appropriately constructed. The ability to write effective, high-level multiple-choice items requires a skill that develops with practice over time. The old adage, "Rome wasn't built in a day" is certainly applicable here. The guidelines in this chapter are designed to give you a head start on the process by pointing you in the right direction for improving your skills for becoming a proficient multiple-choice item writer.

Relevance of Multiple-Choice Items

Assessment of specific learning outcomes must direct the choice of item format. Whatever format is chosen, the items should be specifically designed to elicit knowledge related to the course outcomes at higher-order levels of thinking, as designated by the test blueprint. Multiple-choice items can be designed to address specific content and learning outcomes and are well suited for measuring achievement across cognitive levels.

Documenting that a test is assessing learning outcomes, not trivia, is an essential requirement for establishing content-related evidence of the validity of a test. Every test item should represent course content and a learning outcome. When evaluating a test item, you should first ask, "How does this question relate to the test blueprint?" Only items that directly relate to the blueprint should be included on a test. Another important question to ask is, "Why is this information important for a nurse to know?" Questions that are dubious or inconsequential should be omitted. The multiple-choice format is easily adapted for measuring intended learning outcomes; it is your professional judgment that determines the relevance of individual items for the test.

Item Writing Logistics

In addition to the features mentioned in previous chapters, test development software affords the ability to create professional-looking exams. If you do not have access to this software, the availability of current electronic word processing programs can provide you with the tools to give your classroom tests a professional appearance. There are no longer any excuses for sloppy-looking tests. Carelessness with grammar, spelling, and punctuation reflect poorly on you, the test developer. Additionally, if faculty expect to hold students to high standards on their written assignments, they must hold themselves to even higher standards.

A key requirement for item development is that all faculty members use the same procedure for creating test items. The ultimate goal for every nursing program should be to establish a working item bank. Because consistency is a paramount concern for item bank development, it is beneficial for faculty members to come to a consensus on several key issues at the outset of the item-development process. Chapter 12, "Instituting Item Banking and Test Development Software," thoroughly explains the use of electronic item banking and test development software.

Once the blueprint for a test is agreed upon, faculty members can start writing items. It is a good idea to develop more questions than you need for each area of the blueprint. These "extra" items can be stored in the item bank. Another practical suggestion is to write a few questions each day, particularly after a classroom or a clinical experience when the material is fresh in your mind. Just be careful not to use the same examples that you used to illustrate a point in class, or you will be writing at the recall level. If a particularly interesting illustration of a concept occurs with a group of students, use the experience to write an item and "bank" it for next year.

Style Guide

Consistency of style improves test validity and reliability by decreasing ambiguity, increasing item quality, and engendering student respect for your tests. When all exams in a nursing program follow a style guide, a consistent and professional test appearance is created. Consistency of style also establishes the basis for developing an item bank. It is necessary for all items in a bank to follow a particular style so that they will create a professional impression when they are used together on a test.

A group consensus is necessary for adoption of a test and item-writing style guide. If you use a test development software program, the program will dictate some of these decisions; however, it is helpful to start the process of developing a guide with some suggestions. Basic style suggestions are proposed in Appendix B, "Basic Style Guide." These basic style rules are the ones that I have found to be most conducive to the development of professional-looking and effective multiple-choice items. You will note that all of the items presented in this book follow these style suggestions. Obviously, you should adapt your style to the needs of your individual group. The essential requirement is that a style be followed consistently so that the items look like they are professionally developed and that they belong together when they are used on a test.

Electronic Item Development

Several older texts advocate using 5-by-8 index cards for item development and storage. In this era of electronic word processing, you are wasting your time if you handwrite items and then have them typed onto a test. It is essential that you create your items in an electronic file. If you are not already doing so, start composing your items directly into a word processing program. You will get a much better feel for the item when you see it in typeface, and with very little practice you will be electronically cutting and pasting your way to item-writing proficiency.

Once you have your items in an electronic form, you have established the basis for item banking. Your items will be available for future use. Whether you use test development software or are crafting your items in a word processing program, it is helpful to print each item on an individual sheet of paper for review by your colleagues. Having each item on a separate sheet also facilitates reviewing and sorting the items into a test.

Multiple-Choice Format

The multiple-choice format consists of two parts (see Figure 6.1):

- The *stem*, which identifies the problem or the question

- The *options*, which present the response alternatives. The *key* is the option that is the correct answer, and the *distractors* are the options that appear plausible to the uninformed, but are incorrect responses to the stem.

Multiple-Choice Format

Question

All of these foods are on the lunch tray for a client who is following a low-residue diet. Which one should a nurse advise the client to remove?   } STEM

    A. Chicken noodle soup.   Distractor

    B. Mashed potatoes.   Distractor   } OPTIONS

    C. Broiled flounder.   Distractor

    D. Steamed broccoli.   KEY

Incomplete Statement

All of these foods are on the lunch tray for a client who is following a low-residue diet. A nurse should advise the client to remove the   } STEM

    A. chicken noodle soup.   Distractor

    B. mashed potatoes.   Distractor   } OPTIONS

    C. broiled flounder.   Distractor

    D. steamed broccoli.   KEY

FIGURE 6.1   Multiple-choice format

While the multiple-choice format appears to be very straightforward, item writing is a demanding craft. There are many subtle intricacies involved with developing multiple-choice items that work. Effective multiple-choice items reduce errors by minimizing the possibility of confusing the informed students—and at the same time, minimizing the chance that the uninformed students will guess the correct answer. In this way, effective items increase item discrimination and the overall reliability of the test.

Most faculty members have no difficulty in identifying what they want to test. Many faculty members have difficulty crafting items, however. As with any skill, the more you write the better you become. Following the guidelines presented here will set you in the right direction for developing new items, editing your old items, and evaluating items from textbook item banks. Chapter 10, "Interpreting Test Results," will provide even more direction for improving your items based on item analysis data. Whatever you do, do not throw away your old tests. I have yet to meet a test question that could not be fixed.

Stem Formats

The most important quality of a stem is that it presents a problem that relates directly to a learning outcome. Referring to your learning outcomes every time you develop a stem will ensure that each item is designed to assess the achievement of your course objectives.

Multiple-choice stems can be framed as either a question or an incomplete statement. The most important mechanical aspect of a stem is for it to stand alone; reading the options should not be required to determine what the problem is.

Follow these three basic guidelines to ensure that your item stems are complete:

- Relate the stem directly to a specified learning outcome.

- Include both a subject and a verb in every stem.

- Keep the stem longer than any of the options.

Question

Presenting the stem as a question is the format that many experts prefer for writing multiple-choice items. When the problem is formulated as a question, the item writer is compelled to state the problem clearly and completely in the stem. In real life, when we want a student to solve a problem, we ask a direct question. We do not propose an incomplete sentence and expect the student to finish our thought.

Asking a question is the most direct way to pose a problem. This method of presentation puts a minimum demand on reading skills and ensures that the problem is completely framed in the stem. It also decreases the possibility of introducing grammatical cues with the options. Although a question might require a longer response in the options, a stem that is written as a question is often more effective than framing the stem as an incomplete sentence. Figure 6.2 is an example of a stem presented as a question.

Question Stem Format

Which of these instructions should a nurse give to a client who is taking digoxin (Lanoxin)?

FIGURE 6.2   Question stem format

Completion

In some situations, a stem can be presented more concisely as an incomplete sentence than as a question. The completion format increases the cognitive complexity of the item, however, because students have to rephrase it as a question before responding. This format also requires students to keep re-reading the stem to identify which option correctly completes the sentence. Students lose time when they have to keep reading the stem. This situation poses a particular difficulty for students who speak English as a second language (ESL students) as well as for students who have a learning disability. Remember, the key objective of an achievement test is to identify what a student has achieved in a particular domain. A good item removes all obstacles that would interfere with a student's maximum performance.

While there are arguments against the completion format, they are not sufficient to necessitate that this format never be used. The recommended approach is to attempt to write the stem as a question first; if you have difficulty keeping the problem clear and concise as a question, use the completion format. Make sure that each option completes the stem to form a grammatically correct, complete sentence. The completion format, when used in its proper form, frequently does a better job of clarifying the problem than the question format. Figure 6.3 shows a stem that uses the completion format.

Completion Stem Format

A nurse should monitor a client who is receiving intravenous potassium chloride for side effects, which include

---

FIGURE 6.3   Completion stem format

Item Writing Guidelines

Guidelines and suggestions for developing multiple-choice items have been published by a host of experts in the field of classroom assessment (including, Bower, Linc, & Denega, 1988; Chenevey, 1988; Ebel, 1979; Frary, 1995; Halaydyna, 1997; Haladyna & Dowing, 1989; Kehoe, 1995; Linn & Gronlund, 2000; McMillan, 1997; Mehrens & Lehmann, 1973; Morrison, Smith, & Britt, 1996; Nitko, 1996; Oermann & Gaberson, 1998; Ory & Ryan, 1993; Popham, 1999; Roid & Haladyna, 1982; Schoolcraft, 1989; Trice, 2000; Worthen, Borg, & White, 1993). While there is virtually universal agreement among the authorities in the field that there are no hard-and-fast rules for test development, there is also remarkable overlap and agreement in their suggestions for test and item development.

The guidelines presented here reflect both the suggestions of these authorities and my own experience with developing multiple-choice items that are dependable indicators of student achievement. These guidelines represent the aspects of item writing that are salient enough to be discussed and practiced. It is your own creative touch that you must cultivate and combine with these guidelines to develop your personal item writing style.

The level of detail presented in these guidelines might seem daunting at first. Actually, you will probably find that many of these suggestions reflect basic common sense and will be readily incorporated into your item-writing repertoire. Other suggestions will be easily understood once you actually implement them. Incorporate these suggestions at your own pace. Begin slowly, but get started. You will be pleased that you did.

These guidelines are not rules; rather, they are suggestions. Because testing specialists advocate these guidelines, however, you should seriously consider adopting them. You will find that the quality of your items will improve if you review these guidelines and gradually incorporate them into your own creative item-writing style. You will also find that these guidelines are helpful for item analysis. Chapter 12, "Instituting Item Banking and Test Development Software," discusses methods for using item analysis data to improve items.

General Guidelines

In order to yield reliable and valid results, achievement tests must be direct and meaningful measures of learning that provide students with the opportunity to display the knowledge that they have acquired. The paramount requirement for test reliability is for a test to have well-constructed items, therefore, clarity is essential. Tests are not intended to assess a student's cleverness. We want students to spend test time figuring out the correct answer, not trying to figure out what the question is asking.

If students have attained a learning outcome, a test should afford them the opportunity to demonstrate that attainment. It is unfair if students answer incorrectly because of factors that are extraneous to the purpose of the test. These factors limit and modify student responses and prevent them from showing their true level of achievement. Unfair factors that might prevent students from performing at their best should be eliminated from a test.

A testing situation in itself is anxiety provoking—a factor that we obviously cannot eliminate. While we cannot eliminate the anxiety factor, however, we can take measures to modify it. Students will scrutinize each question for meaning (expressed and implied). Ambiguous items will cause confusion and increase anxiety. Therefore, the precise meaning of every item should be communicated as efficiently as possible. This responsibility puts great demands on the vocabulary and writing skills of the item developer.

Concerns about clarity bring up the issue of reading comprehension. Achievement tests are not tests of reading comprehension. In fact, you should design your achievement tests to be below the reading ability of the students so as not to confound the measurement of reading comprehension with the measurement of skill in the content domain that is being assessed.

In order to compose effective multiple-choice items, the writer must have a mastery of the subject and familiarity with the level of expertise of the students. Suggestions for developing items that promote student ability to demonstrate achievement on a multiple-choice exam include the following:

- Use familiar vocabulary (unless you are testing terminology).

- Keep the items developmentally appropriate; do not include sophisticated higher-level items on an exam for entry-level students.

- Write the test at a reading comprehension level that is below the ability of the students.

- Tailor each item to be read in one minute.

When developing items, you must ensure that each item stands alone. Answering an item correctly should not depend on answering another item correctly. If students miss the first item in a group of connected items, they will miss all subsequent items in the group. A student might well have been able to answer the second question if it were independent of the first item. When answering a question, students should not have to refer specifically to the answer that was given in a previous question, as Figure 6.4 illustrates.

The recommended strategy for developing multiple-choice items is to write the stem and the correct answer first. Then, use the correct answer to model the development of the distractors, and keep the distractors grammatically and contextually parallel to the correct answer. Effective items are written so that the only difference between those who do well on the test and those who do not is the possession of the knowledge that is being measured. These guidelines will help you minimize extraneous differences.

Connected Items

1. A nurse should recognize that a client who has elevated intracranial pressure will most likely receive which of these medications?

    A. Mannitol (Osmitrol).

    B. Digoxin (Lanoxin).

    C. Indomethacin (Indocin).

    D. Nadolol (Corgard).

2. The nurse should plan to monitor the client for side effects of this medication, which include

    A. hyponatremia.

    B. bradycardia.

    C. hematuria.

    D. agranulocytosis.

The answer to item two here is dependent on a correct answer to item one. Therefore, item one has a higher scoring weight on the test. Students who miss item two because they answered item one incorrectly may have been able to answer item two correctly if it had been independent of item one.

FIGURE 6.4   Connected items

An inherent problem with writing stems by using the completion format is that the correct answer frequently provides the most reasonable completion of the stem. You must be careful to write the incomplete statement so that the correct answer and all possible options complete the stem adequately. This problem is not encountered with the question format.

If you use the completion format, make sure that you do not leave a blank at the beginning or in the middle of a stem. As Figure 6.5 demonstrates, this action interrupts the students' reading continuity and makes the stem confusing and difficult to answer. It is much easier to understand a completion stem if the proposed answers are presented as conclusions to an incomplete statement.

Internal Blank

A nurse is caring for a client who has a normal-functioning, double-barrel, transverse colostomy. The nurse should document that the proximal stoma is producing _____ and the distal stoma is producing _____.

Revised

A nurse is caring for a client who has a normal-functioning, double-barrel, transverse colostomy. The nurse should expect the client to have which of these types of drainage from the distal stoma of the colostomy?

FIGURE 6.5   Internal blank

Characteristics of Effective Stems

The stem is the core of a multiple-choice question. It introduces the student to the central problem being posed. Stems should be clear, succinct, focused, and have a positive approach. If the students cannot understand the stem, they will not be able to answer the question. The best stems introduce novel problems for students to solve, rather than paraphrase a textbook (which encourages rote learning).

COMPLETE   The students should understand what the stem is asking before they read the options. After you write a stem, read it alone before you write the options. When reviewing a colleague's questions, cover the options and read the stem alone. If you cannot determine what the stem is asking, it should be rewritten. Figure 6.6 contrasts an incomplete stem with a complete stem. The complete stem poses the complete problem for the student, while the incomplete stem leaves the student guessing what the question might be about to ask.

Incomplete Stem

Steroids

    A. pose a risk for immunosuppression.*

    B. can cause renal shutdown.

    C. increase metabolism.

    D. alter pulmonary function.

Complete Stem

A nurse should advise a client who is taking an oral steroid preparation to report signs of adverse effects, which include

    A. sore throat. *

    B. urinary retention.

    C. weight loss.

    D. dyspnea.

FIGURE 6.6   Incomplete stem

SUCCINCT   Keep your stems clear and to the point. One sentence is not necessarily the best choice. Complex sentences can confuse students. It is better to use two or more sentences if including all of the information in one sentence makes the sentence too complex. The objective is to communicate the problem as efficiently as possible. Students should be able to read and answer each item in less than one minute.

The key to writing effective stems is to specify all of the conditions that are necessary to have the intended response be the only definitely correct answer to the problem while excluding any unnecessary information (see Figure 6.7). Extraneous information increases ambiguity and lengthens the processing time that is required for students to understand what the question is asking.

Diffuse Stem

A 58-year-old accountant has been experiencing substernal chest pressure on exertion for the past six months. He is now admitted to the cardiac care unit for diagnosis and management. Right jugular pulmonary artery and right radial lines are inserted. During the cardiac assessment, the nurse finds that the client has cold, clammy skin, gray skin color, weak rapid pulse, and a blood pressure of 80/50 mm Hg. The nurse most likely interpreted the client's condition to be related to

Succinct Stem

A nurse is assessing a client who is experiencing severe substernal chest pain. The client is diaphoretic, has cold, clammy, gray-colored skin, a weak and rapid pulse, and a blood pressure of 80/50 mm Hg. The nurse should recognize that these client manifestations are most likely related to

The succinct stem decreases the reading time by almost one-half, yet includes all pertinent information. Eliminating extraneous information focuses the student on the problem and makes the item more direct and easier to understand.

FIGURE 6.7   Succinct stem

FOCUSED   Each item should serve one and only one purpose. Therefore, it is important to keep the stem focused on a single problem. Although an item might require a student to progress through a problem-solving sequence, there should be only one problem to solve. If students incorrectly answer a question that includes more than one problem, the teacher will be unable to identify which problem the students missed.

Instructional information in the stem qualifies as extraneous information and can reduce the effectiveness of an item. Irrelevant material that does not contribute to the basis for answer selection will serve only to complicate the reading comprehension of the item. Keep each item focused on the problem at hand, as the focused stem in Figure 6.8 illustrates.

Unfocused Stem

Documentation is a critical component of the nursing process when caring for rape victims. Which of the following entries most accurately represents a woman who comes to the emergency room reporting that she has been raped by a former boyfriend?

Focused Stem

A woman comes to an emergency department and tells a nurse, "I was raped by my former boyfriend." When documenting the event, which of these entries by the nurse most accurately represents the interaction between the nurse and the woman?

The purpose of an exam is to measure knowledge, not to provide instruction. The focused stem eliminates the instructional material and provides a much clearer description of what transpired between the nurse and the woman than the unfocused stem.

FIGURE 6.8   Focused stem

POSITIVE APPROACH   Experts concur that negative stems should be avoided. At the very least, you should always attempt to reword a negative stem positively. The correct answer to a negative stem has to be a false statement. Because students are usually focused on finding correct statements, a negative stem can easily confuse them. In addition, the anxiety generated in a testing situation can cause students to overlook a negative word in a stem. Even when students recognize a negative word, reading time is increased because these stems require a reversal of thought patterns. Figure 6.9 demonstrates how a negative stem can be reworded as a positive stem and demonstrates the effectiveness of the positive approach for framing stems.

Negative Stem

A nurse is assessing a client who has pneumonia. Which of these assessment findings indicates that the client does NOT need to be suctioned?

   A. Diminished breath sounds.

   B. Absence of adventitious breath sounds.*

   C. Inability to cough up sputum.

   D. Wheezing following bronchodilator therapy.

Positive Stem

Which of these assessment findings, if identified in a client who has pneumonia, indicates that the client needs to be suctioned?

   A. Absence of adventitious breath sounds.

   B. Respiratory rate of 18 breaths per minute.

   C. Inability to cough up sputum.*

   D. Wheezing prior to bronchodilator therapy.

FIGURE 6.9   Negative stem versus positive stem

Negative questions are seldom encountered in real practice; therefore, they lack practical relevance. Situations do arise in health care settings, however, where the wrong action can have dire consequences. Use a negative stem only when knowing what not to do is important. Because we do not want a student to miss an answer because of carelessness, be sure to highlight the negative word to alert students to look for the incorrect option.

When highlighting negative words, bold, italicize, and capitalize so that negative words REALLY stand out, as the negative stem in Figure 6.9 illustrates. Only words that reverse the meaning of the stem should be highlighted. Once you start to highlight adjectives and adverbs, such as first, last, most, least, and priority, the impact of highlighting diminishes. Students are then more likely to overlook the emphasis put on the word.

Additionally, highlighting can become very subjective. Faculty will not always agree on what to highlight, and the result will be inconsistent. Students will pick up on the inconsistency and might even argue that they missed a question because you forgot to highlight an adjective or adverb. Keep it simple. Highlight only those words that reverse the meaning of the stem so that the correct answer is the one incorrect option. As long as you explain in the test directions that students should read all options and select the best answer, students will not be placed at a disadvantage.

Qualities of Effective Options

The goal of a well-written test item is to have the stem and options be so clearly written that the informed students, while they are challenged, select the correct option and are not tricked into choosing an incorrect option. At the same time, all of the options should appeal equally to those who are uninformed (the low achievers on the test). When the low achievers choose the correct option and/or the high achievers choose the incorrect option, or if no one chooses a particular option, the test item is not functioning properly.

Keep the options succinct. Long options become a test of reading ability and tend to confuse the reader. If the options are longer than two lines, the problem probably was not fully developed in the stem. As a general rule-of-thumb, keep the options shorter than one line and certainly shorter than the stem.

How many options should be offered in a multiple-choice question? If the distractors are effective, the higher the number the more discriminating the item. Many standardized multiple-choice exams use four options. Good distractors are hard to write, however, and there is no magic in four options. Most importantly, we want to avoid distractors that trick or confuse high-achieving students or that fail to attract low-achieving students. We do not want students to get to the right answer by process of elimination due to the weakness of the distractors.

Four options reduce the chance of guessing, but it is better to use three options if you are unable to come up with a fourth option that is plausible. Having one correct answer and two plausible distractors is better than including a distractor that is implausible just to keep the number of options at four. In fact, if you use three options, you reduce the reading time per question and can include more items on the test.

It is acceptable to include questions with both three and four options on a test. It is less confusing for students and more conducive to face validity to keep all of the items with a uniform number of distractors, however. The major difficulty with four options is that posed with writing distractors. One of the goals of this chapter is to assist you with developing skill in the ability to write plausible distractors.

A key requirement for item plausibility is to have all of the options look alike. Listing the options vertically allows the best visual comparison. They should all be approximately the same length or be listed in ascending length. If one of the options is a disproportionate length compared to the others, as shown in Figure 6.10, it will cause a cuing error in the item. In some cases, it could attract students; in other situations, it could cause students not to select that option. In either situation, a student's choice of an option should not be related to cuing; it should be based solely on knowledge, or lack of knowledge, in the content area.

Disproportionate Option Length

A client says to a nurse, "I have a living will, but I haven't told my family, because I don't want to worry them." Which of these replies would be appropriate for the nurse to make?

A. "You have a right to privacy about this matter."

B. "I won't tell your family, but I have to note it in your chart."

C. "I have to tell your doctor, but I won't tell anyone else."

D. "You should discuss this with your family and doctor so that if a health crisis did occur they would have first-hand information of your wishes so that they could act as you would want them to." *

Option D is disproportionately long, providing a clue to its correctness.

FIGURE 6.10   Disproportionate option length

Another requirement for item options is to place those associated with a value in numerical, chronological, or sequential order. Either ascending or descending order can be chosen. An answer that requires a numerical response will cause confusion if the student has to hunt for the answer. It is much more effective to place such answers in sequential order. Figure 6.11 illustrates the advantage of ordering options.

Disordered Options

A client is to receive quietane (Seroquel) syrup 50 mg po bid. The bottle of Seroquel syrup contains 25 mg per 5 mL. How many milliliters of syrup should a nurse give the client for each dose?

A. 10 *

B. 25

C. 5

D. 20

Reordered Options

A client is to receive quietane (Seroquel) syrup 50 mg po bid. The bottle of Seroquel syrup contains 25 mg per 5 mL. How many milliliters of syrup should a nurse give the client for each dose?

A. 5

B. 10 *

C. 20

D. 25

Notice how the disordered example causes the student to hunt for the correct answer. Keeping the option in order decreases confusion and reading time. Notice also that there are no periods at the end of the options, in order to avoid confusion with decimals.

FIGURE 6.11   Option order

Many test development software programs will scramble options if you want to create different versions of a test. If you want options to remain in a particular order, be sure to disable this feature for the item. If you are storing your items in hard copy, make a notation that the options should not be scrambled.

The more precisely you word your items, the more accurate they will be. Therefore, it is important to provide appropriate labels for answers that relate to values such as vital signs or laboratory values. Figure 6.12 illustrates how labeling values clarifies their meaning and limits student speculation.

Unlabeled Values

Which of these laboratory results should a nurse recognize as suggestive that a client who is diagnosed with schizophrenia has developed an adverse effect of prescribed clozapine (Clozaril)?

A. Blood urea nitrogen (BUN), 16

B. Platelets, 160,000

C. Creatinine phosphokinase (CPK), 55

D. White blood cells (WBC), 3,200 *

Labeled Values

Which of these laboratory results should a nurse recognize as suggestive that a client who is diagnosed with schizophrenia has developed an adverse effect of prescribed clozapine (Clozaril)?

A. Blood urea nitrogen (BUN), 16 mg/dL.

B. Platelets, 160,000 /mm^3.

C. Creatinine phosphokinase (CPK), 55 U/L.

D. White blood cells (WBC), 3,200 μ/l. *

FIGURE 6.12 Labeling values

GRAMMATICALLY CORRECT   Most experts agree that the best approach to item writing is to compose the stem and the key first and then to create the distractors that will parallel the correct answer. It is important to be especially careful about the grammatical structure of all of the options when you use the completion format. Because the correct answer is written with the stem, it usually completes the stem appropriately. It can be all too easy to overlook grammar when you are focused on writing believable distractors. Furthermore, if you change an item after you edit it, be sure to double check the grammatical consistency of all of the options. If only one option is grammatically synchronized with the stem, the students will be inclined to choose it, as the examples in Figure 6.13 illustrate.

Grammatical Inconsistency

When assessing the health needs of a community a nurse should consider that spirituality refers to an

- **A.** participation in an organized religious group.
- **B.** practices and rituals of a particular religion.
- **C.** dimension that is outside the realm of health assessment.
- **D.** individual's beliefs about the meaning of life and death. *

Grammatical Consistency

When assessing the health needs of a community a nurse should consider that spirituality refers to

- **A.** participation in an organized religious group.
- **B.** practices and rituals of a particular religion.
- **C.** a dimension that is outside the realm of health assessment.
- **D.** an individual's beliefs about the meaning of life and death. *

In the inconsistent example the stem is only consistent with the correct answer. This provides the uninformed student with an obvious cue.

FIGURE 6.13   Grammatical consistency

POSITIVE STATEMENTS   As with stems, negativity should be avoided in the options (especially if a negative stem is used). Double negatives cause impossible confusion. Negative options are often used to increase item difficulty. The problem is that they increase difficulty by tricking the students. Negative options are generally not acceptable distractors. Figures 6.14 and 6.15 demonstrate the misleading quality of negative stems.

Negative Options

When physically restraining a client a nurse should consider all of these standards of care EXCEPT

- **A.** obtaining a signed consent from the client. *
- **B.** using the least restrictive device for the shortest time.
- **C.** not keeping restraints on continuously.
- **D.** applying restraints when nonrestrictive alternatives are not effective.

Negative options are particularly confusing when the stem is also negative. Options C & D both include negative terms, which make this question an exercise in logic rather than a true test of knowledge.

Revised

When physically restraining a client which of these standards of care should a nurse consider?

    A. Obtaining a signed consent from the client.

    B. Using the most restrictive device available.

    C. Removing restraints at regular intervals.*

    D. Applying restraints before attempting a nonrestrictive alternative.

FIGURE 6.14   Negative options

Negative Stem With Negative Options

A nurse reviews self-care with a client who has chronic renal failure and an A-V fistula on the left arm. Which of these statements, if made by the client should indicate to the nurse that the client needs FURTHER teaching?

    A. "I will wear my watch on my left wrist." *

    B. "I will not allow anyone to draw blood from my left arm."

    C. "I will not have my blood pressure taken on my left arm."

    D. "I will not carry heavy objects with my left arm."

The word "further" reverses the meaning of the stem so that the student must identify the incorrect option. The "nots" in the options reverse the meaning of the distractors. The correct answer is the only positive one. This is an extremely confusing item!

FIGURE 6.15   Negative stem with negative options

DISTINCT   Each option should be distinct. Retaining as much information as possible in the stem rather than in the responses reduces redundancy and reading time. Words or phrases that have to be repeated in the options should be in the stem, not in the options, as shown in Figure 6.16. The operating principle here is to keep reading time to a minimum.

Another concern with maintaining the distinctness of the options is to avoid overlapping the options. Items should not be partially correct; that is, a correct response should not be part of a distractor. Structuring an item this way confuses students. Keep all of the options mutually exclusive; when options overlap, more than one option may be correct. Figures 6.17 through 6.19 present different applications for keeping options distinct.

Redundant Options

Which of these methods provides a quick estimation of the cardiac rate from the electrocardiogram of a client who has normal sinus rhythm?

A. Count the number of T waves in a five-second strip and multiply by six.
B. Count the number of large squares in an R-R interval and divide by ten.
C. Count the number of small squares between two P waves and multiply by five.
D. Count the number of QRS complexes in six seconds and multiply by ten.*

Revised

In order to obtain a quick estimation of the cardiac rate from the electrocardiogram of a client who has a normal sinus rhythm a nurse should count the number of

A. T waves in a five-second strip and multiply by six.
B. large squares in an R-R interval and divide by ten.
C. small squares between two P waves and multiply by five.
D. QRS complexes in six seconds and multiply by ten.*

The revised item eliminates redundancy and decreases the time needed for reading the question.

FIGURE 6.16   Redundant options versus distinct options

Partially Correct Options

Which is most effective approach for a nurse to take when approaching a suspicious client?

A. Cautiously extend hand.
B. Introduce self and state reason for visit.*
C. Extend hand and state reason for visit.
D. Introduce self and extend hand.

The actions in these options overlap. Including a correct component in a distractor confuses students. Each option should stand alone, with the correct option being the only completely correct answer.

Distinct Options

After introducing oneself, which of these approaches would be appropriate for a nurse to take when initially approaching a hospitalized client who is suspicious?

A. Offer to shake the client's hand.
B. Explain the reason for the visit.*
C. Tell the client that there is no need to be distrustful.
D. Provide the client with a thorough orientation to the facility.

Each of the options is distinct, the distractors contain only incorrect components, and there is only one clearly correct answer. Note that the action of introducing oneself is included in the stem.

FIGURE 6.17   Partially correct options

Overlapping Options

A nurse should explain to a client who is taking lithium (Eskalith) that the dose must be individualized to maintain blood levels between

   A. 0.25–0.5 mEq/L.
   B. 0.5–1.5 mEq/L. *
   C. 1.5–2.0 mEq/L.
   D. 2.0–3.5 mEq/L.

Revised

A nurse should explain to a client who is taking lithium (Eskalith) that the dose must be individualized to maintain blood levels between

   A. 0.15–0.4 mEq/L.
   B. 0.5–1.5 mEq/L. *
   C. 1.6–2.5 mEq/L.
   D. 2.6–3.5 mEq/L.

Each of these options stands alone. One option does not include another.

FIGURE 6.18   Overlapping options

Including One Option Within Another

   A. Affects the client's blood pressure.
   B. Decreases the client's blood pressure.

Option B is included in option A. If B is the correct answer, then A is also correct.

FIGURE 6.19   Including one option in another

HOMOGENEOUS APPEARANCE   In order for options to be equally attractive to students, they all must be parallel in length, grammatical structure, content, and complexity. The more homogenous the options appear, the more challenging the item. Homogeneity refers to appearance only; each of the options must be mutually exclusive, and each one must provide a clear and distinct choice. The correct option must be the only correct option, and the incorrect options must be undeniably wrong. Figure 6.20 shows that the more the incorrect options look like the correct answer, the more difficult it will be for the uninformed students to guess the correct answer.

Opposite options pose a problem in multiple-choice items. If two of the options are opposites, the students will be drawn to decide between those two and ignore the other options. Figure 6.21 shows how opposite distractors can provide a cue to uninformed students.

Heterogeneous Options

Which of these nursing diagnoses would be the priority for this client?

A. Activity intolerance.

B. Constipation.

C. Hypertension.

D. Fluid volume deficit.

Homogeneous Options

Which of these nursing diagnoses would be the priority for this client?

A. Activity intolerance.

B. Constipation.

C. Hyperthermia.

D. Fluid volume deficit.

Option C in the heterogeneous example is not a nursing diagnosis and is therefore inconsistent with the stem and the other options.

FIGURE 6.20   Homogeneous options

Opposite Options

A client has a Sengstaken-Blakemore tube connected to low wall suction. When the client develops respiratory distress, which of these actions should a nurse take?

A. Inflate the tube's esophageal balloon.

B. Deflate the tube's esophageal balloon. *

C. Decompress the tube's gastric balloon.

D. Increase the amount of wall suction.

Distinct Options

A client has a Sengstaken-Blakemore tube connected to low wall suction. When the client develops respiratory distress, which of these actions should a nurse take?

A. Lavage the tube with ice water.

B. Deflate the tube's esophageal balloon. *

C. Decompress the tube's gastric balloon.

D. Increase the amount of wall suction.

In the first example options A and B are opposites, this attracts students to choose between only options A and B and ignore options C and D. By removing the incorrect opposite option, uninformed students are more likely to consider all four options as equally attractive. In addition, in the original question option D is the only option that does not have a "balloon."

FIGURE 6.21   Opposite options

The "Rule of Two Sets" applies to opposite options. If similar structure or wording is included in two options, it must be used in all four options. If two options are opposites, you must use two sets of opposites. As the examples in Figure 6.22 show, two similar options will attract students and cause them to discount the two that are dissimilar, while two sets of opposite options will decrease the guessing ability of the uninformed students.

Rule of Two Sets

One Set of Opposites

A nurse should monitor the client for side effects of the medication, which include

- **A.** hypertension.
- **B.** hypotension.*
- **C.** insomnia.
- **D.** palpitations.

Two Sets of Opposites

A nurse should monitor the client for side effects of the medication, which include

- **A.** tachycardia.
- **B.** bradycardia.
- **C.** hypertension.
- **D.** hypotension. *

In the first example testwise students are apt to ignore options C and D. The second example uses the "Rule of Two Sets" in which two sets of opposites will attract the uninformed student to all four options.

FIGURE 6.22   Rule of Two Sets

Homogeneous options use medical terminology and technical language consistently. If terminology is used in one option, it should be used in all options. Figure 6.23 provides an example of how students will be drawn to choose the answer that appears most technical.

Avoid writing items that have very specific correct answers and very general distractors or very specific distractors with a very general correct answer as Figure 6.24 demonstrates. The students will be attracted to select the option that is different. If one of the homogeneous options in these sets is the correct answer, the question is attempting to trick the students.

SUCCINCT   Succinctness of the options is just as important as succinctness of the stem as Figure 6.25 illustrates. Keeping key words in the stem eliminates repetition in the options. Repeating words in the options causes confusion and unnecessarily complicates the reading of the question. In addition, a distractor should not be partially correct.

Technical Language

A nurse should carefully observe the client for which of these manifestations?

A. Pruritus. *

B. Redness.

C. Bruises.

D. Ringing in the ears.

Revised

A nurse should carefully observe the client for which of these manifestations?

A. Pruritus. *

B. Erythema.

C. Eccymosis.

D. Tinnitus.

Choice A, which is the correct answer, contains the only technical term in the first example. Students are most likely to choose the technical term even if they are not familiar with the material being tested. If B, C, or D were the correct answer in the first example, the question would be a trick item. The revised example uses all technical terms, making the options homogeneous.

FIGURE 6.23   Medical terminology

General/Specific Options

Which of these measures is most important to include when caring for a client during the immediate postoperative period?

A. Repositioning the client at regular intervals.

B. Monitoring the client's cardiovascular status. *

C. Orienting the client to the post anesthesia unit.

D. Checking the client's ability to move the lower extremities.

Testwise students will recognize that the correct answer is the global option.

FIGURE 6.24   General/specific options

Repetitive Words in the Options

Before administering digoxin (Lanoxin) to a client who has congestive heart failure, a nurse should check the client for

    A. bradycardia, hypokalemia, and gastric upset. *

    B. constipation, bradycardia, and hypokalemia.

    C. hypokalemia, dry mouth, and bradycardia.

    D. hypertension, bradycardia, and hypokalemia.

Succinct Options

Before administering digoxin (Lanoxin) to a client who has congestive heart failure, a nurse should check the client for bradycardia, hypokalemia, and

    A. gastric upset. *

    B. constipation.

    C. dry mouth.

    D. hypertension.

In the preceding question checking for bradycardia and hypokalemia are in every option, so they belong in the stem.

FIGURE 6.25   Succinct options

Correct Answer

There should be one and only one correct answer for each question. Perhaps this statement seems too elementary to even mention, but frequently the key is a problem in classroom tests. Whether the correct answer is the only right answer or the best response, the faculty should agree that the designated answer is the only correct one. Writing a referenced rationale for each of your items is the most effective way to assure the veracity of the key. In addition, referenced items can be shared with your students for a very effective test review.

It is critical that the stem specifies all of the necessary conditions that make the intended response the only correct answer. At the same time, you will want to avoid some of the factors that will interfere with the effectiveness of your items. First of all, it is important to randomize the key. The correct answer should be equally assigned to each of the option choices. If you randomize the position of the correct answer when you write the items, it will make it easier to randomize the key when you assemble a test. There should be an equal number of correct answers in the A, B, C, and D positions. Teachers frequently hesitate to assign a correct answer to the A position, and students often assume that teachers prefer the C assignment for the correct answer.

A helpful method for assuring that your key does not become confused is to put an asterisk (*) at the end of the correct option. If you use a test development software program to compose your items, this step is unnecessary because the program will maintain the key once you enter it. If you write your items in a word processing program, however, the key could become confused if you rearrange the options for any reason. Having an asterisk at the end of the correct answer will assure that the key is correct no matter how often you cut and paste your options during test development. You will note that the item examples in this book follow this suggestion.

There are several cues that can "give away" your correct answer to testwise students. These include having a longer and more precise correct answer as compared to the incorrect options, as in Figures 6.10 and 6.26, and phrasing the correct answer in textbook terminology, as in Figure 6.26.

Textbook Language

A nurse should recognize that the manifestations of tuberculosis are related to

- **A.** the production of lymphokine which is stimulated by the immune response to the tubercle bacilli. *
- **B.** a decrease in the white blood cells.
- **C.** an inflammatory response.
- **D.** the increased production of sputum.

Textbook language encourages students to select an option even though they do not understand the material. This option violates two additional guidelines: tubercle bacilli is mentioned only in the key, and the key is much longer than the distractors.

FIGURE 6.26   Textbook language

Designing Effective Distractors

The art of writing effective multiple-choice items requires you to use your creativity and critical thinking skills. Crafting distractors presents the biggest challenge to most teachers. The goal of distractors is to discriminate between the students who are informed and those who are uninformed in the content domain. In order to effectively discriminate, all of the options must be equally attractive to those students who are uninformed.

Distractors should be as attractive as the correct answer to students who have not achieved the desired outcome. If a distractor does not attract students; if the distractors attract the high-achieving students; or if more low achievers choose the correct answer than high achievers, the item is not functioning properly. It takes practice to develop expertise in crafting workable distractors; following the suggestions that follow will help you get started.

One method for increasing the difficulty of a multiple-choice item is to require the student to select the best answer. When you are asking for the one correct answer, the distractors should all be wrong. A question that asks for the "best" answer implies that all of the options vary in degree of correctness, with only one option as the best answer. The difference between these two formats is illustrated in Figure 6.27. Best answer items tend to be more difficult and discriminating than questions that have distinctly incorrect distractors. Items that are written in the best answer format are an effective strategy for developing critical-thinking items. The advantages of this format for writing critical-thinking items are discussed in Chapter 7, "Writing Critical Thinking Multiple-Choice Items."

Best Answer Format

A nurse should give priority to which of these short-term outcomes for a client who is experiencing a panic attack?

    A. The client will have decreased symptoms of anxiety.

    B. The client will avoid frightening situations.

    C. The client will learn thought-stopping techniques.

    D. The client will remain safe during the episode. *

Each of the options is a possible outcome, while option D is clearly the priority outcome at this time.

Correct Answer Format

Which of these questions would be appropriate for a nurse to ask when assessing a client for bulimia?

    A. "How many times a day do you eat?"

    B. "For how long have you been at your current weight?"

    C. "Do you have particular food dislikes?"

    D. "Do you ever eat in secret?" *

In this example all of the distractors are incorrect. Only D is an appropriate answer. Because there is only one correct answer, the stem cannot ask for a best answer, such as, "Which of these questions should a nurse ask first?"

FIGURE 6.27 Best answer format

PLAUSIBILITY   It is not enough for a distractor to be wrong; it must be plausible without being tricky (see Figure 6.28). If high-achieving students chose distractors because they are tricky, the item loses its usefulness. At the same time, highly implausible or absurd distractors contribute nothing to the effectiveness of a test. Ideally, all of the incorrect options should appeal only to the uninformed student. The uninformed student should be not be able to eliminate the incorrect options with certainty. Learning to write plausible distractors takes practice.

Implausible Distractors

A nurse should recognize that which of these individuals is most likely to have a personality disorder?

A. An 18-year-old man who is beginning a new relationship and is unsure as to whether he is ready for a long-term commitment.

B. An 24-year-old woman who is unable to show emotion, has no friends, and is estranged from her family. *

C. A dependable, loyal 30-year-old man who expresses himself through art.

D. A 43-year-old woman who describes herself as shy and reticent.

Options A, C, and D are implausible while option B is so obviously correct.

FIGURE 6.28   Implausible distractors

COMMON MISCONCEPTIONS   You probably have lots of ideas for plausible distractors right at your fingertips. Keep a log of the common misconceptions that students have in clinical practice. Make a list of classroom questions that students frequently ask. Common errors and beliefs of students translate into very believable distractors. Figure 6.29 shows how common misconceptions can be translated into effective distractors.

Common Misconceptions

When a client has a seizure which of these actions should a nurse take?

A. Place a spoon in the client's mouth.

B. Protect the client's head.*

C. Restrain the client's extremities.

D. Insert an airway into the client's trachea.

This item recognizes that students who are not familiar with the content will be drawn to the common misconceptions identified in the distractors.

FIGURE 6.29   Common misconceptions

RELATED STATEMENTS THAT DO NOT APPLY   A statement that relates to a situation that is close to the question but does not satisfy the requirements of the question at hand will attract the uninformed students. Students who have not mastered the content will remember hearing or reading these facts but will be unable to correctly apply the information. A related statement that does not apply to the stem requires the students to make a judgment related to the accuracy of the statement as well as its relevance, as Figure 6.30 illustrates.

Related Statements That Do Not Apply

A client who has congestive heart failure says to a nurse, "I really don't understand what is wrong with my heart." Which of these explanations would be appropriate for the nurse to give to the client?

- **A.** "There is a blockage in the arteries that supply your heart muscle."
- **B.** "Your heart is having difficulty pumping an adequate blood supply for your body." *
- **C.** "The impulses that direct the beating of your heart are acting randomly."
- **D.** "There is a bulging in the major vessel that leaves your heart."

While A, C, and D are responses that describe cardiac pathology, they do not apply to CHF. They will look familiar to the uninformed student. Writing distractors that correctly explain another situation is much more effective than "creating" pathophysiology, such as: "The blood is moving too rapidly through the left side of your heart."

FIGURE 6.30   A related statement

SEEKS HELP APPROPRIATELY   Items that call for the nurse to seek assistance require the student to recognize when a situation requires the expertise of another health care professional. Because students hesitate to select the option "Call the physician," it makes a very poor distractor. When that option is the correct one, however, it works well because it requires the student to carefully discriminate among the alternatives to recognize when a situation requires the attention of the physician. You might prefer to have the nurse take an action in the stem first, but calling the physician is an acceptable format, as the question in Figure 6.31 demonstrates.

Seeks Help Appropriately

A client who has esophageal varices develops hematemesis. In addition to checking the client's pulse and blood pressure which of these actions should a nurse take?

- **A.** Obtain a specimen for blood gas analysis.
- **B.** Increase the client's oral fluid intake.
- **C.** Administer the client's prescribed lactulose (Cephulac).
- **D.** Notify the client's physician. *

FIGURE 6.31   Seeks help appropriately

YES, NO WITH EXPLANATION   The item in Figure 6.32 requires a two-step reasoning process. The yes/no explanation format requires students to recognize not only the correct answer, but also the reason for the correct answer. These items tend to be difficult with high discrimination indices if they are written following the guidelines presented in this chapter.

Yes, No With an Explanation

A client who has insulin-dependent diabetes mellitus (IDDM) is taking both insulin injection (Regular, Humulin R) and isophane insulin (NPH). A nurse identifies that the client is taking the insulin as two separate injections each morning. Should the nurse advise the client to change this procedure?

   A. No, regular insulin is unstable and, therefore, should be given separately.

   B. Yes, mixing the insulins in one injection decreases the use of injection sites. *

   C. No, NPH will be altered if it is mixed with regular insulin.

   D. Yes, because giving the two insulins in one injection prevents errors in dosage.

FIGURE 6.32   Yes, no with explanation

Characteristics to Avoid

Cues are irrelevant and unintended clues to the correct answer. Cues enable students to make the correct response without having the required ability. Cues will negatively impact the reliability of a test. An effective multiple-choice item eliminates these cues so that students are only able to answer the question correctly if they have the knowledge that the question requires. Grammatical inconsistency and homogeneity are two cues that were previously discussed. It is obvious that violating many of the guidelines presented in this chapter will provide cues to the uninformed student. Several additional cues will be identified in the section to follow. Your goal as an item developer is to avoid these cues to ensure that your items contribute to the test.

VERBAL ASSOCIATIONS   Repeating key words from the stem only in the correct option provides a cue to testwise students. Verbal associations connect the correct answer to the stem, as is seen in Figure 6.33.

Verbal Association

A nurse should recognize that the first step in resolving an ethical dilemma related to a client's advanced directives is to

   A. recognize that an ethical dilemma exists. *

   B. identify the moral point of view of the client.

   C. assess the viewpoints of all involved parties.

   D. determine the client's health status.

The word "ethical" is repeated only in the correct answer.

FIGURE 6.33   Verbal association

QUALIFYING WORDS   Qualifying words provide cues to students because they neutralize the option, making it a safe choice. Words such as often, seldom, sometimes, usually, and generally are most often found in the correct answer, as shown in Figure 6.34. These words qualify the key by indicating that the option does not have to be true all of the time. Testwise students recognize that if one option is not definitive, it is the safe choice. If you use qualifying words, keep the options homogeneous by including qualifiers in all of the options.

Qualifying Words

When screening a group of senior citizens for hypertension, a nurse should understand that elderly clients who have hypertension

    A. often have no symptoms. *

    B. will refuse to accept treatment.

    C. have an underlying cause for the problem.

    D. respond more positively to medication than younger clients.

The qualifying word in the correct answer provides a clue because the option is more general. The key allows that some clients will have symptoms, while the distractors are absolute.

FIGURE 6.34   Qualifying words

SPECIFIC DETERMINERS   Words such as never, none, all, and always are specific determiners. These words are the antitheses of qualifiers. They indicate that a situation is absolute. Because very few things in nursing are absolute, using specific determiners only in the incorrect answers will provide a cue to testwise students, as Figure 6.35 shows. Specific determiners are seldom used in the correct answer, and testwise students are aware of this fact. These words are appropriate to use in the stem; however, they should be used sparingly in the options and then only when they can be appropriately used in the correct answer. Items should be written to test more than a student's ability to recognize that unequivocal statements are seldom true.

Specific Determiners

When planning care for an elderly client who is bedridden, a nurse should recognize that pressure ulcers

    A. always result from the client's inability to ambulate.

    B. develop when tissue is subjected to sustained pressure. *

    C. can always be prevented by vigorous massage.

    D. will never develop if the client is well nourished.

Specific determiners rule out the possibility of an exception to the rule. The rule "never say never" applies here. "Pressure" is also a cue in the stem.

FIGURE 6.35   Specific determiners

ALL OF THE ABOVE   All of the above and none of the above are used most often when a teacher cannot think of a fourth option. All of the above is particularly helpful to testwise students who are able to select the correct answer based on incomplete information (refer to Figure 6.36). These students recognize that if they can identify two correct answers, then all of the above is correct; or if they can identify that one answer is incorrect, then all of the above is incorrect. The use of all of the above should be avoided; it is much more effective to rephrase the question so that four plausible alternatives are provided.

All of the Above

When assessing a client who reports having sleep deprivation, a nurse should assess the client for manifestations, which include

- **A.** confusion.
- **B.** slowed response time.
- **C.** diminished reasoning skills.
- **D.** all of the above. *

The testwise student need only recognize that two of the options are correct to identify that the correct answer is "all of the above." Therefore, a student who has incomplete understanding can guess the correct answer.

FIGURE 6.36   All of the above

NONE OF THE ABOVE
None of the above should be used sparingly, if at all. After all, if there is no correct answer to the question, why ask it in the first place? Figure 6.37 clarifies how the use of none of the above as a distractor produces an ineffective item.

None of the Above

Which of these components of the nursing process determines the extent to which the planned client outcomes have been achieved?

- **A.** Assessment.
- **B.** Planning.
- **C.** Evaluation. *
- **D.** None of the above.

Testwise students know that they should avoid the none of the above option, which reduces the plausible options to three.

FIGURE 6.37   None of the above

Some experts advocate the use of none of the above to decrease the chance of correctly guessing when the student must perform an operation to obtain the correct answer. Several authorities acknowledge the benefit of using this option when testing calculations in a multiple-choice format (Ebel, 1979; Linn & Gronlund, 2000; Mehrens & Lehmann, 1973; Nitko, 1996; Popham, 1999).

The use of none of the above is recommended only when students are more likely to answer the question and then look at the options, such as with a math calculation as shown in Figure 6.38. Students might be able to estimate the correct calculation answer on a multiple-choice exam. When you want to be confident that students can perform the calculations, use none of the above so that students will not be able to assume that the correct answer is included in the options. This alternative avoids giving clues to students when their incorrect solution is not among the options. When none of the above is an option, the students have to be certain that their solution is correct. Without none of the above as a choice, it is easier to guess without really knowing how to calculate. There is one caution to remember, if you use none of the above as an option: the correct answer must be absolute. The answers for math calculation questions, for example, cannot be rounded up or down. Unless you specify in the stem that the answer is approximate, a rounded number is not absolutely correct and none of the above is the technically correct answer, even when you intend another option to be the correct answer. If you choose to use the none of the above format for math calculation items, reserve it for answers that are absolute, such as the example in Figure 6.38.

None of the Above

A nurse is preparing to administer 2 mg of a medication to a client. The medication is available in a vial that is labeled 1 mg/0.5mL. How many milliliters should the nurse administer to the client?

   A. 0.5

   B. 1.5

   C. 2.0

   D. None of the above. *

In this example the student must be sure of the answer to recognize that none of the above is correct.

FIGURE 6.38   None of the above math

A problem with the none of the above option is that students might not believe that this option is ever correct. If students do not believe that it is a viable choice, it will not work as an option. It is important to explain to students who are not used to the inclusion of the none of the above option on a test that this choice will sometimes be the correct option.

MULTIPLE-MULTIPLES   The goal of item development is to make the question as clear as possible and to eliminate any extraneous factors that would confuse students. Multiple-multiple or complex multiple-choice items directly contradict this goal. The example in Figure 6.39 shows just how confusing a multiple-multiple item can be. This item format is unnecessarily complex and is more a test of a student's logic ability than a direct and meaningful indicator of a student's achievement.

Multiple-Multiple

A screening test for a disease is found to have a sensitivity of 90% and a specificity of 95%, which means that of the people who had the test

- **A.** 5% of those who have the disease were identified as positive.
- **B.** 95% of those who do not have the disease were identified as negative.
- **C.** 10% of those who were identified as negative have the disease
- **D.** 90% of those who were identified as positive do not have the disease.

   - **A.** A & B are true and C & D are false.
   - **B.** C & D are true and A & B are false.
   - **C.** A & C are true and B & D are false.
   - **D.** B & C are true and A & D are false. *

This question is impossibly confusing. Even if the student can interpret the stem, an inordinate amount of time is needed to decipher what is being asked.

Revised

A screening test for a disease is found to have a sensitivity of 90% and a specificity of 95%. A nurse should interpret this as meaning that of the people who had the test

- **A.** 5% of those who were identified as negative do not have the disease.
- **B.** 10% of those who have the disease were identified as positive.
- **C.** 90% of those who were positive do not have the disease.
- **D.** 95% of those who do not have the disease were identified as negative. *

FIGURE 6.39   A multiple-multiple item

TRICK ITEMS   Trick items are designed by item writers who are under the false impression that any means of increasing item difficulty is acceptable (refer to Figures 6.40 and 6.41 for examples). The problem is that these items will trick both low and high achievers, and the item will not be an effective indicator of student achievement. These items lure students to second-guess themselves and to select an incorrect answer because of an extraneous cue. Students become understandably distrustful of faculty members who employ tricks in their tests.

Trick Item

A client who is receiving an intravenous infusion develops dyspnea and increased blood pressure. A nurse should recognize that which of these problems may be developing?

A. Infection.

B. Air embolism.

C. Fluid overload. *

D. Hypovolemia.

This question will confuse students. It is a trick item because while an embolism is not associated with elevated blood pressure, it is definitely associated with dyspnea. The inclusion of dyspnea in the stem will mislead students. The question would be more effective if it included several clear manifestations of fluid overload and/or if air embolism was left out of the distractors. Even the most experienced professional would not make a definitive diagnosis based on two manifestations. In addition, it is far more important to ask what a nurse should do when a client experiences an untoward reaction to an intravenous infusion.

FIGURE 6.40   Trick item

Trick Item

Which of these client manifestations would support a nursing diagnosis of fluid volume deficit?

A. Tachycardia. *

B. Decreased respiratory rate with prolonged expiratory phase.

C. Dysuria.

D. Diaphoresis.

Students may be drawn to select B because it is the longest answer. Figure 6.10 illustrates a disproportionately long correct answer which provides a cue to students. This example violates the same rule, but it is particularly unfair because it purposely tempts the student with a cue to the wrong answer.

FIGURE 6.41   Another trick item

HUMOR   Humor is an indispensable tool in the classroom. It is out of place on an exam, however. While humor can decrease tension in the classroom, it can have the opposite effect in a testing situation—particularly with highly anxious test takers (Haladyna, 1997). Students who do not "get" the joke on a test can become embarrassed and distracted by laughter during a test. ESL students in particular will have difficulty understanding the humorous intention of an item and can lose their focus when trying to interpret the meaning of such an item (Klish, 1994). Consider how distracting it would be to have students around you laughing during an exam while you are struggling to decipher what a question is asking. In addition, using a humorous option decreases the number of plausible distractors and will make the test artificially easier. Haladyna points out that humorous questions might encourage students to be less serious about taking the test (1997). The best approach is to save your humor for classroom instruction.

Item Rationale

An effective method for increasing the validity of your multiple-choice items is to write a rationale for each question. A quality rationale includes a textbook reference and explains why the correct answer is correct and also why each of the distractors is incorrect. This explanation should be kept with the item in an electronic file, either in an item banking program or in a word processing file. Writing rationales for your items not only increases the quality of the items and ensures the veracity of the key, but it also provides a valuable resource for student test review.

Question Difficulty

While it is important not to trick or confuse students, it is just as important to present them with questions that challenge them and that are trustworthy measures of their abilities. Chapter 3, "Developing Instructional Objectives," reviews the cognitive levels and notes that the levels of knowledge, comprehension, analysis, and application are particularly suited to the development of multiple-choice items. Item writers should strive to develop items at the higher levels of application and analysis. In fact, very few items at the knowledge and comprehension levels should be used on a nursing exam. Appendix C, "Targeting Cognitive Levels for Item Writing," provides lists of verbs and examples of items at the different levels of cognitive ability.

The questions on the NCLEX-RN are written as four-option, multiple-choice items at the cognitive levels of knowledge, comprehension, application, and analysis. The majority of questions are written at the application and analysis levels (NCSBN, 1997, p. 3). The *National Council Detailed Test Plan for the NCLEX-RN Examination* is a very informative booklet that was developed to provide content direction for item writers for NCLEX. This document organizes subcategories according to the phases of the nursing process and includes specific activity statements from the job analysis after each client needs subcategory. The *Detailed Test Plan* demonstrates how the job analysis is linked to the test plan (Steele & Wendt, 1999) and is a very valuable resource for faculty to use in item writing.

An item writer can manipulate the difficulty of items. The important principle is that the difficulty of the item should relate to the content and instructional objectives being measured, not to the use of vocabulary. Keeping distractors homogenous increases the difficulty level of the question because students have to make fine distinctions. Using the best answer approach also increases the difficulty of the item.

Framing Questions in Terms of the Nursing Process

Using the nursing process as a framework for item development poses several advantages for crafting quality multiple-choice items. In addition to increasing face validity of the test, it increases the pertinence of the questions that you ask. If you have to put a nurse and/or a client in every stem, you have to think about the relevance of the question for nursing practice. This approach helps to eliminate trivial items from your tests.

Another advantage of the nursing process approach is that it promotes the development of unique situations in which to frame nursing problems. While nursing process questions can be written at all of the cognitive levels, the format encourages item development at higher levels. Novel situations can be designed that require students to analyze and/or apply information, rather than to simply recall facts.

It is clear that the nursing process format is viewed as a valuable framework for item writing. The items on NCLEX-RN themselves are written in terms of the nursing process. While the 1995 NCLEX-RN test plan (NCSBN, 1995) actually included the phases of the nursing process equally in the blueprint, the current plan (NCSBN, 1998) states that it integrates the nursing process across the categories of client needs.

Following the example of the NCSBN in developing your items makes perfect sense. The nursing process format is viewed by the NCSBN, one of the most respected test developers in the country, as a valuable method for framing items that address nursing concerns. Following the lead of the experts when writing items to assess the content and objectives of your course is a logical approach to improving the quality of your multiple-choice exams. Figure 6.42 provides definitions of the phases of the nursing process that can be used to guide the development of multiple-choice items.

Item Shells

Appendix D, "Sample Item Stems for Phases of the Nursing Process," provides suggested item stems that are framed in the context of the nursing process. These stems are successful items with their content removed, hence the term "item shell." Substitute your content, and your stem is written. The challenge of writing the correct option and several plausible distractors still remains, but these stems will set you in the right direction for writing items within the nursing process context that assess higher-order thinking. Using this format will also help you focus on writing items that test material of importance, rather than the recall of trivial facts.

While stems are useful as prompts to get you started with developing your own items, do not mistake them for templates for all item writing. It is important to have variety in the structure of items on a test; we do not want all of the questions to be too similar. Use the stems as a starting point for developing your own item writing strategy.

Peer Review

Item review by your colleagues is critical for developing effective test questions. Chapter 5, "Implementing Systematic Test Development," addresses the need for blueprint review, and item review is equally important. A relevant blueprint will designate what the items on the test should address. It is the teacher, however, who must ensure

Stages of the Nursing Process

Assessing: Obtaining, confirming, and communicating data about a client.

Analyzing: Selecting relevant data and drawing inferences and conclusions to identify potential and/or actual problems that require nursing assistance. Includes identifying nursing diagnoses and communicating results of analysis.

Planning: Making plans with the client and family to set goals and establish outcomes to deal with the identified problems. Includes prioritizing and communicating plan.

Implementing: Includes actions, such as communicating, teaching, performing or assisting with activities of daily living, and informing client and/or family about health status in order to achieve the established outcomes.

Evaluating: Gauging the client's response to the planned actions, and the movement toward or away from identified goals. Determining the extent to which client outcomes have been achieved.

FIGURE 6.42 *Stages of the nursing process*

that the items actually meet the requirements of the blueprint. The relationship of each item to the content domain must be verified in order to assure that the test actually represents the content.

In addition to verifying that the items meet the blueprint, item review involves editing and determining whether the items meet the guidelines presented in this chapter. Circulating items among colleagues for opinions and suggestions is a helpful method for addressing blueprint issues and improving item quality. Omit the answer key from the items. If an expert in the content area is unable to answer the question, it most certainly needs revision. The objective is not to find fault or criticize but only to critique the items based on agreed-upon criteria in order to increase the quality of the items. The questions in Figure 6.43 summarize the guidelines presented in this chapter. Use these questions as a guide for critiquing multiple-choice items.

Allowing an adequate time frame for blueprinting and item development increases the likelihood that the items will address the test plan. It is unrealistic to expect members of a teaching team to devote adequate time to editing and carefully examining the relevancy of test items on short notice. In fact, you will not be able to do a careful job of analyzing items yourself if you do not allow enough time.

Item Review

Does the item reflect the principles of item development?

Overall:

Does the item reflect a learning outcome established for the course?

Does the item deal with an important aspect of the course content?

Is the item testing information that is important for a nurse to know?

Is the item succinctly worded?

Does the item stand on its own?

Does the item contain any cues?

Is the meaning of the item clear?

Does the item contain any spelling or grammatical errors?

Is the item original (not a direct textbook quote)?

Is the item written at an appropriate reading level?

Does the item address higher-level cognitive ability?

Does the item follow the style guide agreed upon by the faculty?

If the guidelines are not followed, is the item effective?

The Stem:

Does the stem address a learning outcome of the course?

Does the stem present a single, clearly formulated problem?

Is the problem clearly stated in the stem without reading the options?

Does the stem provide all the necessary information to solve the problem?

Is the stem clear without extraneous information?

Does the stem use the nursing process format?

Is the stem stated so that there is one, and only one, correct answer?

Is the stem phrased to avoid repetitive words in the options?

If the stem contains a negative word, is it unavoidable and ***HIGHLIGHTED***?

The Options:

Do the options overlap?

Are the options homogeneous?

Is there only one correct answer?

Are options placed in logical order?

Are distractors incorrect, yet plausible?

Are all distractors completely incorrect?

Has the position of the correct answer been randomly placed?

Are all of the options grammatically correct and consistent with the stem?

FIGURE 6.43 Criteria for item review

Summary

Expertise in multiple-choice item writing is an ability that develops with practice over time. Because quality test items are essential for the validity and reliability of your classroom exams, you need to develop this expertise. This chapter is designed to provide you with direction for becoming a proficient item writer. These guidelines are related only to the mechanical aspects of the item writing process that can be discussed and practiced, however. While they provide important direction, your creativity and clinical expertise are just as important to successful item writing. In order to write valid and reliable multiple-choice exams, you need to cultivate your expertise in both aspects of the process. Chapter 7, "Writing Critical Thinking Multiple-Choice Items," specifically addresses how to call upon your creative abilities when writing critical thinking items, and the chapters that follow provide additional guidance to assist you with objectively analyzing and improving your item writing ability.

7 Writing Critical Thinking Multiple-Choice Items

> *"Man's mind stretched to a new idea never goes back to its original dimensions."*
>
> —Oliver Wendell Holmes

Critical thinking is a complex process. Consequently, assessing critical thinking ability is a complex process that presents a unique challenge to nursing faculty. While the guidelines for multiple-choice item development that are presented in Chapter 6, "Developing Multiple-Choice Test Items," form the essential basis for creating critical thinking multiple-choice items, that is only the beginning of the process. Writing critical thinking multiple-choice items requires that you think critically yourself; that you call on all of your own reasoning and creative skills to assist you in assessing the behaviors that represent the characteristics of critical thinking in your students.

Characteristics of Critical Thinking Items

Multiple-choice items can play an important role in a multifaceted approach to the assessment of critical thinking. In order to effectively contribute to that assessment, multiple-choice items must be focused on measuring higher-order thinking ability; recall and comprehension items cannot effectively assess the cognitive processes associated with critical thinking. Item development at the application and analysis cognitive levels is the basic criterion for the measurement of critical thinking. This criterion applies to all formats of critical thinking measurement instruments. It is of particular concern in the development of multiple-choice items, however, because it is so convenient to write these items at the recall and comprehension levels.

While the ability to address higher-levels of cognition is a key attribute of effective critical thinking multiple-choice items, it is certainly not the only requirement. An appreciation of the characteristics of multiple-choice items that support their ability to assess critical thinking will assist you in developing these items successfully.

Sequential Reasoning

Although the retention of information is required to determine the solution to a critical thinking problem, it is the ability to use the information in a unique situation that distinguishes a critical thinking multiple-choice question from an item requiring lower-level cognitive skills. Recall- or comprehension-level questions will not tap the abilities that comprise critical thinking skills. As the recall question in Figure 7.1 illustrates, questions at the lower levels call for rote memorization. Students are called on to choose from the proposed options based on recollection; they are not required to solve a problem.

Recall Question

The dose of intravenous heparin should be adjusted to maintain the client's activated partial thromboplastin time (APTT) at how many times the control?

- A. Less than 1.5
- B. Between 1.5 and 2.5 *
- C. Greater than 2.5 and less than 3.5
- D. Between 3.5 and 4.5

This question simply requires the student to recall that the client's APPT should be between 1.5 and 2.5 times the control.

FIGURE 7.1   Recall question

Sequential reasoning requires more than just simple recognition; it is a process of deliberation that requires at least two logical steps. Critical thinking multiple-choice items that are written at the cognitive levels of application and analysis, require students to use sequential reasoning to solve the problem presented by the question. Appendix C, "Targeting Cognitive Levels for Item Writing," presents suggestions for applying cognitive levels to item writing. This guide is a valuable tool to assist you in developing your multiple-choice items so that they meet the basic criterion for critical thinking assessment: measuring the application and analysis levels of cognition. Be careful not to confuse the cognitive level of *analysis* with the nursing process phase of *analysis*. While questions related to the analysis phase of the nursing process are frequently written at the cognitive level of analysis, items can be written at the cognitive levels of analysis and application for all phases of the nursing process.

A critical thinking item requires students to draw on their nursing knowledge, to approach the problem from more than one viewpoint, and to apply concepts in order to select from among the alternatives the one that proposes an appropriate, or the most appropriate, solution to the problem. Figure 7.2 illustrates how the recall question in Figure 7.1 can be translated to an application question.

Application Question

A client who is receiving intravenous heparin has an activated thromboplastin time (APTT) of 2.5 times the control. In addition to documenting the finding, which of these actions would be appropriate for a nurse to take?

   A. Call the lab for a stat repeat of the test.

   B. Discontinue the client's heparin infusion immediately.

   C. Continue to monitor the client. *

   D. Alert the blood bank to have a unit of packed cells available.

This question takes the recall question of Figure 7.1 one step further. In addition to asking the student to recognize that the APTT should be between 1.5 and 2.5 times the control for a client who is receiving heparin, it requires the student to apply that information. Notice that the question calls for the student to select an "appropriate" action from among "these" actions. This critical thinking item does not assume to include the universe of all possible options. In this question, while the client's APTT is within the range, it is at the top of the range. The nurse could also check the client's vital signs, or observe for adverse effects, such as hematuria. However, the question asks the student to discriminate among the options offered, and only one of these is appropriate.

FIGURE 7.2 Application question

Language

Notice that in the example in Figure 7.2 the student is required to select the option that proposes an appropriate solution, not the only solution. Note the wording of the stem: "Which of *these* actions would be *appropriate* for a nurse to take?" There usually is more than one approach for solving a problem in nursing. A critical thinking multiple-choice item does not purport to present the only answer to a problem; rather it requires the student to select the appropriate answer from the options presented. The phrasing, "Which action should a nurse take?" indicates that there is only one way to approach the problem. Students could argue that they have solutions that are not included in the options that are as reasonable as the one proposed.

It is acceptable to use more definitive wording when the correct answer is also definitive, particularly when the distractors represent incorrect interpretations of the data, or if you are asking students to prioritize the provided alternatives. Although it is best to avoid the word "should" when the list of options does not include the universe of possible answers, "should" can be appropriate in situations where a nurse is clarifying information, collecting and/or interpreting data, prioritizing diagnoses or interventions, or evaluating outcomes. However, as Figure 7.3 illustrates, it is always important to include the word "these" in the stem because you are asking the student to select from the list of options that is presented, not from the universe of alternatives.

Evaluate Outcomes

A client who has hypovolemia is receiving an intravenous infusion. A nurse should identify that the infusion is having the desired effect if the client develops an increase in which of these assessments?

    A. Thirst.

    B. Heart rate.

    C. Urine output. *

    D. Pulse pressure.

This critical thinking item requires the student to recognize the desired outcome of intravenous therapy for hypovolemia and then to identify which of the proposed responses would indicate that therapeutic response. The stem correctly uses "should" because the student is asked to interpret the data that is presented. There is only one correct answer. There are not degrees of correctness among these alternatives, the distractors are all incorrect. Note that while there are additional assessments that could indicate a successful outcome, such as increased blood pressure, the nurse is not deciding which action to take; the nurse is interpreting the data at hand from among "these" alternatives.

FIGURE 7.3   Evaluate outcomes

A critical thinking multiple-choice item calls on the student to use critical thinking skills to distinguish between the options proposed to select which of the responses would be appropriate for the situation presented. It may seem very picky and technical to take such exacting construction precautions when writing these items. However, when you call on students to use critical thinking skills to solve a multiple-choice item, you do not want to have any words in the item that could distract the students or cause them to "read into" the question.

Figure 7.4 and Figure 7.5 provide two more examples of how you can translate a recall question into a critical thinking multiple-choice item.

Best Answer Format

In Chapter 6, "Developing Multiple-Choice Items", the "best answer" format was introduced. This format is particularly suited to the development of critical thinking multiple-choice items because higher-level cognitive skills are required to determine which alternative is the "best," the "first," the "priority," or the "most important." Remember, it is necessary that all of the options vary in degree of correctness with one being the best answer. If the distractors have no element of correctness then do not use the best answer format.

With this format, shown in Figure 7.6, the student must first use sequential reasoning to solve the problem and then must differentiate between the degrees of correctness of the proposed options to determine which is the correct answer.

Recall

A nurse should monitor a client who has had a thyroidectomy for signs of

A. laryngeal nerve damage. *
B. increasing intracranial pressure.
C. carotid artery distension.
D. hypercalcemia.

Application

Which of these nursing measures should be carried out at regular intervals when caring for a client during the immediate post operative period after a thyroidectomy?

A. Asking the client to speak. *
B. Checking the client's pupillary response.
C. Palpating the client's carotid arteries.
D. Instructing the client to flex and extend the neck.

Instead of asking for simple recall this question asks the students to understand the potential complication and plan measusres for early identification of the problem.

FIGURE 7.4   Recall translated to application

Recall

A nurse is aware that a screening test has high specificity. This means that the test

A. provides precise findings.
B. correctly identifies those who have a disease. *
C. accurately identifies those who do not have a disease.
D. has a high correlation with severity of disease.

Analysis

A nurse who is planning a health screening program identifies that a particular screening test has a specificity of 90%. The nurse should recognize that this indicates that the test accurately identifies

A. 10% of those who actually have the disease.
B. 10% of those who do not have the disease.
C. 90% of those who actually have the disease. *
D. 90% of those who do not have the disease.

Rather than asking for recall of a definition, this item asks the student to interpret findings based on an understanding of the definition of the term. Note that the revised item also presents two sets of opposites.

FIGURE 7.5   Recall translated to analysis

Best Answer

A nurse plans all of these measures for a client who was rescued from a fire and has deep burn injury of the chest and arms. To which of these measures should the nurse assign priority during the emergent phase of burn management?

A. Monitoring the client's respiration. *

B. Assessing the client's peripheral circulation.

C. Measuring the client's urine output.

D. Preventing the client from developing infection.

This question requires the student to identify the treatment plan for a client who has a burn injury. The student must identify the threat to the airway from this type of injury in order to discriminate between degrees of correctness among the options to select the best answer.

FIGURE 7.6 Best answer critical thinking item

Novel Problems

A critical thinking multiple-choice question must propose a novel problem for the student to solve. Even if an item appears to be at a high cognitive level, if the students are familiar with the problem, the question is a recall item. For this reason, only the teacher really can determine the true cognitive level of an item.

If you use a situation as an example in class, you cannot convert it to an item and use it on a test for the same group of students. If you translate a situation that occurred in the clinical setting with a group of students into an item, you cannot use it on a test with that group of students. This is not to say that you should not use real-life experiences as models for test items. You certainly should. Just be careful that you bank those items for exams that will be given to a group of students who have not been exposed to the situation.

The more unique the situation in a question, the more its solution will involve the use of critical thinking skills. A familiar or textbook situation requires only that the students use recall. Unique situations require that students analyze and synthesize information to determine a course of action, as Figure 7.7 illustrates.

Applying Learning Outcomes

It is essential for the validity of a test that the items measure the objectives and content of the course as designated in the test blueprint. Valid critical thinking items reflect your definition of the construct, the objectives you established to measure student achievement, and the content domain as specified by the blueprint. It only makes sense to use the learning outcomes that you painstakingly developed at the beginning of the test development process to frame your critical thinking multiple-choice items. Applying the specific behaviors that define the learning outcomes as the basis for item development is critical for ensuring that your items are measuring critical thinking as it is reflected in your definition.

Unique Situation

An elderly client is about to have a minor surgical procedure. The client says to a nurse, "I really don't know why it is so important for me to have this surgery." The nurse notes that the client has signed a consent for the surgery. Before administering the client's preoperative medication, which of these actions would be appropriate for the nurse to take?

A. Discuss nonsurgical treatments with the client and document the discussion in the client's medical record.

B. Reassure the client that this is minor surgery and the surgeon has an impeccable reputation for performing only surgery that is beneficial for clients.

C. Contact the client's adult children to determine if they understand the need for the surgical procedure.

D. Inform the surgeon that the client does not understand the need for the surgery. *

This situation introduces several factors which make it unique: the client is elderly, the procedure is minor, the consent is already signed, and the client is not yet medicated. The question requires the student to analyze the information to identify the important principle. Note that none of the information is extraneous. All of the information in the stem works to establish a unique situation and each of the options relates to the stem.

FIGURE 7.7   Unique situation

Because they operationalize the characteristics of critical thinking, the specific behaviors that define the learning outcomes can easily be adapted to form the basis for critical thinking multiple-choice questions in the content domain specified by the blueprint. It is important to note that the focus on assessing critical thinking should not diminish the significance of the content domain. Remember, the blueprint is a two-way grid. In order to meet the blueprint specifications, the questions must be framed to assess critical thinking in the content domain specified in the instructional course.

Refer to the tri-level critical thinking objective from Table 4.2. The learning outcome of "Demonstrating Sensitivity to Context" is operationalized by five specific defining behaviors. The examples that follow for each of the specified defining behaviors illustrate how they can be translated into effective critical thinking items:

- Asks relevant questions (see Figure 7.8)

- Solicits the client's perspective (see Figure 7.9)

- Identifies situations requiring modification (see Figure 7.10)

- Establishes priorities for the individual's situation (see Figure 7.11)

- Verifies the value of the plan to the client (see Figure 7.12)

These examples illustrate how each of the specific behaviors that define and provide evidence for a learning outcome lends itself to the development of critical thinking multiple-choice items that directly measure that outcome. Employing these behaviors for item development will provide the basis for construct-related evidence of validity for your classroom exams and will increase your confidence in the results of these exams.

Asks Relevant Questions

A community nurse is visiting a client who has congestive heart failure. The client has gained four pounds in the last week and has lower extremity edema. Which of these questions would be appropriate for the nurse to ask?

   A. "Do you realize how dangerous it is for you to go off your diet plan?"

   B. "How have you been following your treatment plan this week?" *

   C. "Did you forget to take your medicine this week?"

   D. "Weren't you concerned enough about the swelling in your feet to call me?"

Only answer B seeks to investigate the reason for the change in the client's condition. The nurse is attempting to gather data before determining the cause of the problem. In answers A and C, the nurse has already decided what the cause is. Answer D is inappropriate, it criticizes the client for not reporting the situation.

FIGURE 7.8   Asks relevant questions

Solicits the Client's Perspective

A client who has borderline hypertension says to a nurse, "My mother had high blood pressure and she died from a stroke." Which of these responses would be the most appropriate one for the nurse to make initially?

   A. "We have more effective medications to control your blood pressure today."

   B. "Your hypertension may be controlled with lifestyle modification."

   C. "How carefully did your mother follow her treatment plan?"

   D. "You seem concerned about the health risks associated with hypertension."*

While options A, B, and C are based on correct statements, they do not seek the client's perspective, in fact they dismiss the client's concerns. Only the correct answer, option D, seeks to explore the client's perspective.

FIGURE 7.9   Solicits the client's perspective

Identifies Situations Requiring Modification

A client is in the post-anesthesia unit after having a transurethral prostatectomy with epidural anesthesia. The client has a Foley catheter attached to continuous bladder irrigation and is receiving an intravenous infusion of 5% normal human serum albumin (Plasbumin) solution. A nurse should initiate immediate action if the client

A. reports having low back pain. *

B. has a pulse oximetry reading of 92%.

C. is unable to move the lower extremities.

D. has clots draining in the bladder irrigation fluid.

This question requires the student to analyze the situation to identify which client response requires intervention and which are acceptable findings.

FIGURE 7.10   Identifies situations requiring modification

Establishes Priorities

Which of these nursing actions is the priority when a client who has a fever of unknown origin is to be started on intravenous antibiotic therapy?

A. Review the client's white blood cell count.

B. Ensure that the client's blood culture sample is drawn. *

C. Obtain the client's body temperature.

D. Increase the client's fluid intake.

With this best answer critical thinking question, the student is required to evaluate the correctness of the options. While all of the options are appropriate actions, B is the priority.

FIGURE 7.11   Establishes priorities

Verifies the Value of the Plan to the Client

A client who has lung cancer has agreed to attend a group session to stop smoking. After three meetings with the group the client says to a nurse, "This will never work. I cannot stop smoking." Which of these responses would be appropriate for the nurse to make?

A. "Give the group a little more time, you have really just begun."

B. "Are you receiving support outside of the group, particularly from your family?"

C. "Should we explore a different approach to assist you to stop smoking?" *

D. "Are you really telling me that you want to continue smoking?"

"One size does not fit all" when planning client care. Only option C considers the client's value of the plan, the distractors do not attempt to obtain client input for plan development.

FIGURE 7.12   Verifies value of plan to client

Critical Thinking and the Nursing Process

An effective approach for writing items to assess critical thinking in nursing is to develop them in the framework of the nursing process. As Chapter 6, "Developing Multiple-Choice Items," points out, using the nursing process model increases the relevance of the question for nursing practice and also promotes the development of novel situations.

The stems in Appendix D, "Sample Item Stems for Phases of the Nursing Process," provide a useful foundation for writing critical thinking multiple-choice items. Appendix F, "Relationship of Critical Thinking Characteristics to the Nursing Process," delineates how each critical thinking characteristic relates to the nursing process. If, for example, you want to develop a question that assesses whether a student can delegate responsibility appropriately, you can look in Appendix F and locate the defining behavior "Delegates Responsibility Appropriately" under the learning outcome, "Demonstrates Sensitivity to Context." The table indicates that this behavior relates to the planning and implementation phases of the nursing process. You can then refer to Appendix D for stems under either the planning or implementation phase of the nursing process to write an item that measures the ability to delegate responsibility appropriately.

Figure 7.13 presents a planning question that measures the ability to prioritize when delegating responsibility.

A nurse is planning staff assignments. Which of these clients would be the most appropriate one for a nurse to assign to a nursing assistant?

A. A 24-year-old client who had an appendectomy four hours ago.

B. A 45-year-old client who is receiving intravenous heparin.

C. A 65-year-old client who is receiving inhalation therapy for acute asthma.

D. A 78-year-old client who had a hip fracture repair three days ago. *

FIGURE 7.13   Planning item/Delegates responsibility appropriately

Summary

Producing critical thinking items is a challenge. The guidelines from the previous chapter provide the framework, and the learning outcomes, which were established at the outset of the course, provide the natural basis for critical thinking multiple-choice item development. It is your own creativity and critical thinking skills that are needed to translate the specific behaviors that define these outcomes into items that assess higher-order thinking in the content domain as specified in the test blueprint. This chapter builds on the basics presented in the previous chapter and moves forward with direction and examples to help you improve your ability to create and evaluate critical thinking multiple-choice items.

While providing you with direction for developing critical thinking multiple-choice items, this discussion also reinforces the need for a comprehensive approach to the assessment of critical thinking. Although well constructed multiple-choice exams can provide useful assessment information, there is certainly a need for a variety of approaches for assessing this complex construct, as Table 4.4 illustrates. Students should be able to reason out their own solutions to complex questions, and it is important that faculty provide them with a variety of opportunities to do just that. The essential point is to recognize the valuable role that multiple-choice items can play in a systematic multifaceted approach for the assessment of critical thinking learning outcomes.

8 Assembling, Administering, and Scoring a Test

"Be prepared, be sharp, be careful, and use the King's English well."

—Robert N. C. Nix

If you have been following the guidelines proposed in this book, you have put a great deal of time and effort into crafting your exam. You have carefully developed a blueprint based on your objectives and outcomes and you have painstakingly written, edited, and reviewed items. You have made this effort to create a valid and reliable instrument that will provide you with trustworthy evidence of student learning. However, you are not finished yet! The final steps are just as important as the initial procedures for establishing the validity and reliability of your test results.

The goal of every test is to provide students with an opportunity to demonstrate their best performance. The processes of assembly, administration, and scoring of a test can influence student performance and introduce measurement error that will affect the validity and reliability of your test results. A systematic approach to these processes will reinforce that the test is functioning as you intended (Linn & Gronlund, 2000).

Assembling a Test

Once your items are written, edited, and reviewed for relevancy to the test blueprint, you are ready to assemble the test. Teachers often have the misconception that the design phase of test development is a simple clerical task. In fact, if careful attention is not devoted to the process of assembling a test, much more time will be spent correcting mistakes after the test is duplicated or even worse, administered. A well planned,

133

systematic test assembly process helps to avoid errors that could affect students' scores (Gaberson, 1996).

The final appearance of your test is important for establishing the reliability and validity of the interpretations you will make based on the test. While a professional appearance lends face validity to your exams, tests that are illegible, carelessly word-processed, or collated incorrectly introduce measurement error. Poorly designed tests confuse and annoy students, increase their test anxiety, and give the impression that you have carelessly prepared the exam. Teachers expect students to use care when completing written work. In fact, some teachers deduct credit from students who submit sloppy work or who have grammatical or spelling errors in their written work. Teachers should hold themselves to an even higher standard than the one to which they hold their students. Remember, nothing you write will be more carefully scrutinized than your exams.

Arranging Items

Printing each item on a separate sheet facilitates the sorting and arranging of test items. Each sheet should have space for the item, the rationale, the instructional objective, the learning outcome, and the content measured by the item. Having items on separate sheets not only provides flexibility for assembling the test, it also facilitates item retrieval for editing, revision, and entry of item analysis data after the test.

If you use a computer test development program, the program will keep track of all of the items with their data, and will also provide you with a printout of whatever information you request. The software will sort and arrange the items by whatever criteria you require. One of the important features of test development software is that the item and its accompanying data are never separated.

If you must manage your items in a word processing program, it is essential to establish a system to ensure that the items do not become separated from their data. Storing your items on individual pages in a word processing program will help you to keep track of your data and will make it easier for you to import your items into an electronic item bank once you begin using this software. Chapter 12, "Instituting Item Banking and Test Development Software," discusses the advantages of test development software to electronically manage this process.

When sorting items for a test, group items together that have the same format. This is not an issue if the test consists entirely of one item format type, such as multiple-choice. However, if you include more than one format type on the same test, such as an essay or short answers with multiple-choice, be sure to keep all of the items of the same type together with a specific set of directions preceding each item group of the same format.

Consider the key when arranging items. You do not want the correct answer to be the same letter for more than three questions in a row. Nor do you want a letter to be omitted as the key for several consecutive items. Students pay attention to the key; they even refer to it for clues to the correct answer. Because you do not want students to be misled by the pattern of a key, have the correct answer evenly distributed among all the possible letter options.

It is not advisable to move the location of a correct answer in an item to solve the problem of randomizing a key. The distractors should be left in the position assigned to them by the item writer. As you remember from Chapter 6, "Developing Multiple-

Choice Items," there are strategies associated with ordering options. In addition, manually reordering options increases the potential for introducing error into the key. Instead of reordering the options, consider the letter representing the correct answer as one criterion when organizing the items on a test. Some test development software programs attempt to decrease cheating by scrambling the order of the options to create different test forms. If you want different test forms, but do not want the order of your options scrambled, select a software program that enables you to scramble the order of the items while maintaining the order of the options. In any event, avoid manually reordering the options of an item.

Experts generally agree that items on a test should proceed from easier to more difficult (Linn & Gronlund, 2000; Nitko, 1996). This arrangement helps to decrease anxiety and frustration and has a motivating effect on students. Even well prepared students can become anxious when confronted with difficult items at the beginning of a test. Starting an exam with easier items builds confidence and gives students the opportunity to answer the initial items quickly while reserving extra time to analyze the more difficult questions (Oermann & Gaberson, 1998).

If it is not possible to arrange every item on the test in ascending order of difficulty, you should at least start the test with several of the easier items. Students who encounter very difficult items at the beginning of a test can become discouraged. In fact, they may even spend excessive time laboring over these difficult items and run out of time before they reach items at the end of the test, which they would have been able to answer. If you are creating multiple forms of a test by scrambling item order, be sure to keep the first few items the same for every form so that every student encounters the same easier items at the beginning of the exam.

When including items on a test, it is important to have a range of difficulty level for each content area and objective on the test. For example, a test that includes all of the difficult items in one content area and all of the easy ones in another content area would not provide valid results. Because all of the blueprint categories are important, even if they are weighted differently, it is important to distribute the difficulty levels across the questions that are included in each category.

If you use test development software, manipulating the test items is as simple as clicking your mouse. If your items are in a word processing program, you will need to "cut and paste" them to create the test. Remember to keep track of the data that is included on the page with the item in the word processing program when you "cut and paste." Using test development software or the "cut and paste" option, means that there is no longer any need for a test to be "typed." Once your items are developed, they can be copied easily from the testing or word processing program where they are stored. Figure 8.1 summarizes the key points for arranging the items on a test.

- Print each item on separate sheet

- Group items of the same format together

- Randomize the key

- Start the exam with easier items

FIGURE 8.1   Arranging items on a test

Editing and Proofreading

Professional test developers not only have expert panels to review their blueprints, items, and assembled exams, they also employ experienced word processors and professional editors to ensure that their tests are "polished" before they are published. Although classroom teachers do not usually have these resources, it is important that your tests have a professional appearance for face validity. Poorly edited tests reflect on you. They tell the students that you do not care or that you lack the competence to write clearly and correctly.

There is nothing more distracting or anxiety provoking than to have to make several corrections on the blackboard at the beginning of a test, or to have students raising their hands during an exam to point out typographical errors or omissions. Chapter 6, "Developing Multiple-Choice Items," reviews the principles for ensuring that your items are grammatically correct and consistent. It is also important to carefully review the whole test once it is assembled. Exams that have a professional appearance convey the message to students that quality is important in both teaching and testing. Therefore, it is imperative that every teacher who produces a test carefully reads the test once it is assembled.

Before giving the test to an editor, print a final copy, and take the test yourself. This enables you to key the test and check for errors. If you do not have an editor, call on the expertise of your colleagues. After you have taken and reviewed the test, provide your colleagues with an unkeyed test copy to edit and proofread, and ask them to answer the questions as a final check of the clarity of the items.

The final version of the test should also be carefully read for spelling, punctuation, and grammatical errors. Make sure the test "hangs together;" that the style and formatting are consistent and that all of the questions are written in the present tense. Discrepancies can creep in, especially if different people write the items.

It is also important to check the test for cueing. Cueing within items was discussed in Chapter 6, "Developing Multiple-Choice Items"; cueing can also occur when one question gives away the answer to another. In addition to giving away the correct answer, cueing can also lead students to choose the incorrect answer by misleading them. To eliminate cueing, look for the same or similar options in two items that are near each other. Check to see if an option is the correct answer for one item and is repeated as the incorrect answer for another nearby item. Inspect the items to determine if one provides the answer for another. Examine the questions to make sure that two of them are not asking the same thing. Tests that are developed by more than one person, such as in an integrated nursing exam where adult and pediatric questions are on the same test, are especially prone to cueing. When items cue each other, one item may have to be removed from the test, or the two items may have to be separated in the test. Figure 8.2 summarizes the key points for editing and proofreading a test.

- Allow adequate time
- Take the test yourself
- Inspect for spelling, punctuation, and grammatical errors
- Examine for consistency of style and formatting
- Check that all questions are written in the same tense
- Analyze for cueing

FIGURE 8.2 Editing and proofreading a test

Formatting

There are several technical issues that are related to formatting items on a test. The best approach is to develop a uniform format for all the nursing courses in a program and then to take the time to check that each test follows this format. This not only gives a uniform and professional appearance to all the exams, but it also facilitates the transferal of items from one course to another when content adjustments are made between courses.

There are several widely accepted suggestions for formatting a test. First, you should allow for adequate room for each item on the page, with a double space between items. Then, number the items sequentially throughout the test and list their answer options in a vertical column under the stem with each option preceded by a letter. There are numerous examples of formatted items that follow this template in Chapter 6, "Developing Multiple-Choice Items:"

   1. Question or Incomplete Statement

      A. First option

      B. Second option

      C. Third option

      D. Fourth option

Make sure that the stem and options are kept together on the same page and that margins are available for the students to use for marking items to revisit. And never, yes I said never, have items printed on two sides of a page. This practice can cause confusion and distraction for the students, particularly if the stem is on one side of a page and the options are on the other. If your institution requires that tests be copied on both sides of a page, first protest, and then, if you are unsuccessful, allow your students extra time to complete the test, and be extra careful to keep all the stems on the same page as their associated options.

Note, it is very important that you check and recheck your exams for proper formatting, and any editorial and proofreading changes before submitting them for copying. Taking the time to carefully review the test before it is reproduced will facilitate a seamless process on exam day and will ultimately improve the reliability of your exams. Refer to Figure 8.3 for a summary of the key points for test formatting.

- Develop a uniform format
- Allow a double space between items
- Number items sequentially throughout the test
- List options vertically under the stem
- Precede each option with a letter
- Keep each stem with all options together on the same page
- Provide margins on each page
- Print the exam on ONE side only of a page
- Double check the formatting before copying

FIGURE 8.3 Formatting a test

Providing Directions

A good test is not only a well-planned collection of items; a good test includes a set of rules that must be made clear to students. Clear test instructions are essential for students to be able to demonstrate their maximum ability. If directions are not understandable, the test will not accomplish its purpose.

Students should be told about any special directions before the day of the test. They should know what materials are allowed, such as calculators or scrap paper; they should know what will be excluded from the testing room, such as cell phones or electronic pagers; and they should know what they are required to bring to the test, such as pencils or student identification. Print the directions for the test on a cover sheet so that the students can refer to them during the test. A cover sheet prevents students from reading the questions while you are distributing the tests, and it helps them to focus when you read the directions out loud. Also provide space on the cover sheet for the students to print and sign their names. A signed cover sheet facilitates the tracking of tests for added security, and it enables you to locate an individual's test should any questions arise after the exam.

Directions for multiple-choice exams should not be elaborate, but should include at least these points:

1. **Basis for scoring**   Identify how many items are on the test and how much credit will be given for each correct response. Explain if any items are included for extra credit. If your test includes more than one item format, advise the students of this at the beginning of the test and group the individual formats together in separate sections. Print specific directions and the basis for scoring immediately before each individual test section.

2. **Time limit for the test**   Explain the time constraints for the test in the written directions. In addition, after reading the test directions out loud, announce the exact times that the test will begin and end. Assure your students that ample time is available for completing the test. It is usually helpful to announce to students when half of the allotted time has elapsed. However, in order to avoid creating stress by surprising students, it is important to tell students at the beginning of the test that you will be making a "time-remaining" announcement. It may also be beneficial to periodically write the time remaining on the classroom backboard. Time is a major concern for students. In order to reduce their anxiety, be sure that students understand exactly how you will be communicating the time remaining to them. In addition, it is most helpful to have a large wall clock in the test room.

3. **How to select answers**   Inform students whether they are to select the "best" answer or the "correct" answer. It is also crucial to ensure that students clearly understand how their answers should be recorded on the scannable form. Pay special attention to directing students to keep track of their responses. If they skip a question, they need to have a system to ensure that they do not fill in an answer in the wrong spot on the answer sheet.

   In addition, advise the students to use caution with erasing. Many students have the tendency to "second guess" themselves, which can result in changing a correct answer to an incorrect one. Advise the students that they should change an answer if they feel confident that their initial selection was incorrect, but caution them against making changes based on guessing. If students do change an answer, remind them to carefully erase all traces of their first choice.

4. **Consequences for guessing**   Explain to students whether they will lose credit for incorrect answers. Correction for guessing is sometimes used on standardized tests. However, it is not usually recommended for classroom tests because these tests are already subject to much more measurement error than standardized tests. If you choose to use a scoring program that allows you to correct a student's score for guessing, make sure that the students understand exactly what the implications are for guessing.

The test cover sheet in Figure 8.4 includes all of the criteria for a complete cover sheet with test directions. Use it as a model for developing a cover sheet for your exams.

Answering the questions listed in Figure 8.5 will ensure the thoroughness of your final review of a test.

Reproducing

Reproducing involves yet another time issue! Most likely your support staff handles the task of reproducing the tests for you. If your situation is similar to that of most educational institutions, support staff are stretched to their limit. Plan ahead. You want a professional outcome, so allow staff enough time to reproduce the tests. Reproduction should be completed several days before the test.

Before you submit a test for copying, be sure that the master is exactly the way you want it. Carefully check that all items are there, that they are numbered consecutively, and that the pages are in order. Ask your staff to make a sample copy from the master to check if the contrast is suitable and the quality is acceptable. Set the copier to collate and staple the copies if these features are available. If hand collating is required, extra careful checking of the final copies is essential. Remember to make sure your staff is aware that the test is to be copied on one side only and that enough copies are produced; one for each student and several extras for the examination proctors.

Most paper-and-pencil exams today are scored with a scanner. This frees up a teacher's time and also facilitates the generation of test and item analysis. Students must record their answers to tests that are scanned on a separate sheet, or scannable form, that is compatible with the scanner. Make sure that the scannable form uses the coding (letters or numbers) for the answer options that corresponds to the coding used on the test. Students can become confused if, for example, you labeled the question option letters A through D and the scannable answer form uses number 1 through 4 for the option choices.

Once the tests are reproduced, each test should be numbered and an answer sheet should be marked with the same number. The answer sheet should then be inserted under the cover sheet of each test. This assures that each answer sheet can be matched to a test booklet and provides a security control for the tests and answer sheets.

SCHOOL OF NURSING

FUNDAMENTALS OF NURSING CARE
EXAMINATION I
FALL 2000

Keep this test booklet closed until the proctor tells you to start the test.

This is a **closed book** test that consists of **50 questions**. Each question is worth **2 points**. You have **60 minutes** to complete the test. Do not refer to your text or notes. Calculators must be checked by the proctor. No other electronic devices are allowed in the testing room.

Select the **one** option that **best** answers each question. There is **one correct answer** for each question. There is **no penalty** for guessing. Do not waste time on a question that you find difficult. Skip it and return to it when you have finished the test. Avoid wild guessing. Use the knowledge you have to **answer every question**, even when you are not perfectly sure of your answer.

Follow These Directions Carefully:

- Check that your test has 14 pages in the correct sequence.
- Use only a **#2** pencil.
- Remove the scantron answer sheet that is inserted in this booklet, and fill in the identifying information in the top left hand corner.
- Check to be certain that the exam number on your answer sheet matches the number on your test booklet.
- Circle the one correct answer to each question in the test booklet.
- Darken the circle on the answer sheet that corresponds to the one correct answer for each question.
- Be cautious with changing answers. If you do change an answer, erase your first mark completely on the answer sheet.
- If you skip a question, make sure to keep your place on the answer sheet.
- Mark any question that you skip in the test booklet so that you can easily return to it.
- Stay in your seat until you receive permission to leave it.
- If you have a question during the test, or if you finish the test before the time is up, raise your hand and a proctor will come to you.
- When the exam is over, put your pencil down and wait for the proctor to collect the test materials from you.
- Sign and print your name on the lines below.

Signature: _____

Print Name: _____

FIGURE 8.4   *Sample cover sheet with directions*

- Does the test appear professional?

- Are the test directions clear, complete, and accurate?

- Does the test start with easier items?

- Are the difficult items distributed across the blueprint categories?

- Is the key accurate?

- Is the key randomized?

- Does each item stand alone?

- Does any item cue another item?

- Do any of the items overlap in content?

- Does each question test information that is important for a nurse to know?

- Does each question represent the content and instructional outcomes of the course?

- Do the items follow the style guidelines agreed upon by the faculty?

- Is the test printed on one side of a page?

- Is the test free from typographical, spelling, and grammatical errors?

- Is the test formatted correctly, with adequate margins, and clear, legible font?

FIGURE 8.5 Guidelines for a final test review

Maintaining Security

Safeguarding the security of the test is the teacher's responsibility from the time the items are developed until the test is scored and destroyed. Every faculty members must be responsible to carefully guard electronic and hard copies of the item bank. Just as you would never leave a copy of your personal bank statement in a lunchroom, or fax a copy of it to a public mailroom, the test bank should be treated as a confidential document. If the security of the item bank file is violated, the items are useless.

Another important concern is where to store the tests during the time between reproduction and exam day. A securely locked closet is the simplest solution; just be certain that the exam administrators have access to the closet on exam day (and students or other interested parties do not!). Additional considerations include the security of the copy room and the trash from the copy room. How secure is your test disposal facility? Should you shred exams before disposing of them?

While these questions and concerns may seem extraordinary to some of you, others will relate to the extreme measures that desperate students will take to obtain copies of exam questions. It is critical that only authorized personnel have access to the test. If a student gains access to the test, the results will lack validity and reliability. By taking a few simple precautions, you can save yourself a lot of trouble.

Administering a Test

Conditions surrounding the administration of a test are another potential source of measurement error. The main goal of administering a test is to provide students with a fair opportunity to demonstrate their achievement of the learning outcomes. Fair assessment requires that you provide a test-taking environment that is conducive to the students' best efforts, while minimizing factors that introduce measurement error. A systematic approach to the administration phase of the testing process will limit the problems that can interfere with the reliability and validity of your test results. As with all phases of the test development process, the key factor is to plan ahead.

Physical Environment

Make sure ahead of time that the environmental conditions of the physical space assigned for the test are appropriate. The room must have sufficient seating, light, and ventilation, and be large enough for adequate spacing between desks. The test environment should also be free from noise and interruptions. If the room is subject to distracting noise, such as from construction work, ask for a room assignment change. Minimize all interruptions by posting a sign on the door to the room stating that a test is in progress. You cannot eliminate all distractions, but planning ahead will keep them to a minimum.

Several days before the exam, make sure that the tests are ready and do a final count. On the day of the exam, arrive at the testing room at least 30 minutes before the starting time. Arrange the seating to maximize the distance between students. In situations where you are concerned about students sharing information during a test, you may want to assign seats. Assigning seats is one of the most effective deterrents for cheating. If you have a small number in the class, an easy method for seat assignment is to put "post-it" notes with student names on each desk, or to cut up a student roster and tape each student's name to the assigned seat.

While seat assignment can be complicated for large lecture groups, it is even more important for deterring cheating than with small groups. One approach is to post the seating diagram outside the classroom and assign seats by number to students. Another suggestion is to seat the students randomly by having them "draw" their seat number before the test. Whatever method you choose, assigning seats is recommended as the most effective impediment for student cheating.

Psychological Environment

When students are excessively anxious during a test, they are not able to demonstrate their maximum performance. Linn and Gronlund (2000) identify several teacher behaviors, which can increase test anxiety, and therefore should be avoided:

- Using tests as a threat or punishment: "If the grades on this test are poor, you can expect the next test to be even more difficult."

- Giving dire warnings: "This is the most important test of the semester."

- Stressing time limits: "You have to work fast to finish this test on time."

- Emphasizing the consequences of failure: "If you fail this exam, you will not be able to proceed in the program."

It is the teacher's responsibility to motivate students to do their best in every testing situation. A positive approach focuses students on their abilities. You can establish a positive psychological environment for students by preparing them for the test in advance, and by using these guidelines to offer them well-developed, fair tests. When students perceive that a test is a fair assessment, test anxiety is reduced.

Clear instructions that are positively focused help to reduce anxiety. Keep the negative words in the directions to a minimum. Emphasize what the students should do, and avoid focusing on what they should not do. Consider Figure 8.6. While both of these directions convey exactly the same message, which one is more conducive to reducing student anxiety? It is obvious that the negative approach sets up an adversarial student-teacher relationship at the very outset of the test. If you communicate in a positive manner, your students will perceive that you consider them to be responsible learners. You will boost their confidence and reduce test anxiety.

Positive: Keep this booklet closed until the proctor tells you to start the test.

Negative: Do not open this booklet until you are told to do so.

FIGURE 8.6   Positive versus negative directions

While it is important for you to recognize your role in reducing test anxiety, it is just as important for students to recognize that the best antidote for test anxiety is to be well prepared for an exam. Students must be responsible for their own learning. The guidelines presented in this book help you to communicate that message from the outset of a course. When students accept the challenge of attaining the learning outcomes of a course and they are given a fair opportunity to demonstrate that attainment, their anxiety will be reduced to a healthy level. Student motivation is enhanced if you clearly communicate to them throughout the semester that although you are there to facilitate the learning process, they must achieve their own success.

Academic Misconduct

While it is critical that student performance is not hampered by the testing environment, preventing the environment from falsely enhancing student performance is equally important. Twenty-two years ago Ebel noted, "Cheating on examinations is commonly viewed as a sign of declining ethical standards or as an inevitable consequence of increased emphasis on test scores and grades" (1979, p. 185). Unfortunately, cheating remains all too common on college campuses today. Whatever the cause, cheating is not only ethically wrong, it poses a serious threat to the validity of the inferences made from your exams (Cizek, 1999).

Cheating affects all students. While the dishonest student may receive an inflated grade by cheating, cheating has a negative effect on the honest student. Those who do not cheat are placed at a disadvantage for grades, scholarship awards, graduate school admission, and employment positions (Cizek, 1999). All the effort that goes into developing a measurement instrument is worthless if cheating occurs on an exam, because cheating ruins the reliability and the validity of a test. Therefore, teachers have an obligation to discourage cheating and to report it when it does occur. An ounce of prevention is invaluable here. Careful planning of classroom tests can counteract the various methods that students use to cheat.

When students perceive testing as a fair opportunity to demonstrate their achievement, the incidence of cheating is reduced. However, it is very naive to assume that your students will not cheat just because you have painstakingly developed an exam to meet the criteria outlined in this book. The stakes are very high in nursing education and you will be doing a disservice to the honest students if you do not take measures to discourage cheating.

You have to be proactive to counteract cheating. Procedures must be established to maintain test security during the preparation, assembly, reproduction, storage, administration, and scoring of the test. Several of the procedures specified for choosing and preparing the physical environment for a testing experience will also decrease the opportunity for student cheating. Having students sign the cover sheet, using identification numbers on the tests and answer sheets, and assigning seating are all measures that will counteract cheating.

CHEATING STRATEGIES   In order for you to be able to establish specific strategies to prevent cheating, you must be aware of the methods that students use to cheat on classroom exams. Cizak (1999) identifies many of the cheating schemes that students use. These strategies include:

- Arranging to sit near friends
- Sharing information stored in cell phones or calculators
- Using sign language or signals to communicate with each other
- Dropping answer sheets on the floor in the view of others
- Leaving one's seat to ask a question of the proctor, while surreptitiously observing the answers of others
- Using a "cheat-sheet," written on tissues or hidden in places such as a necktie, skirt hem, pocket, and so on
- Having another student take the test
- Diverting a proctor's attention so that others can cheat
- Using a microrecorder to record questions for others
- Photographing questions with a micro camera to share with others
- Removing test material from the room to share with others
- Neglecting to turn in an answer sheet and claiming it was lost

DETERRING CHEATING   Students have devised countless innovative methods to give and receive information before, during, and after a test. These strategies are sometimes impossible to detect or prevent. The best defense is a good offense. The most effective method for preventing cheating is to have an adequate number of vigilant proctors. Two proctors are the minimum for every group testing situation; it ensures that the students are not left alone if one proctor has to leave the room. Ideally, there should be at least one proctor for every twenty students. Have additional proctors if you have a reason to be concerned. Once students realize that you are serious about preventing cheating, they will be hesitant to risk the consequences of cheating.

It is your responsibility to make cheating impossible. Consider these procedures, consolidated from the suggestions of several experts, to deter cheating (Airasian, 1997; Cizek, 1999; Ebel, 1979; Gaberson, 1996; Linn & Gronlund, 2000):

- Establish a clear testing procedure in the syllabus and in the test directions.

- Have a clear, enforceable policy regarding cheating.

- Use an adequate number of proctors, who are fully aware of the test administration procedure. A minimum of two proctors is essential.

- Require that proctors be fully attentive to supervising students—not reading or involved in any other activity. Proctors should establish eye-to-eye contact with students as they circulate through the room.

- Produce more than one form of the exam. Even if you have only one form, label the cover sheet as if there are two or more forms. Let the students think that there is more than one form.

- Arrive early and assign seats before the test. Cheaters try to sit together. Most cheating occurs when students can select their own seats.

- Provide adequate space between seats. Use alternate seats if possible.

- Require students to leave all books, notes, bags, and extraneous clothing at the front of the classroom. Students should not be allowed to wear hats, sunglasses, and so forth.

- Do not allow students to bring notepaper into the testing room. Provide the students with scrap paper if they are not allowed to write in the test booklet.

- Prohibit students from sharing materials such as pencils, erasers, and calculators during the test.

- Check all calculators and ban all other electronic equipment from the testing room.

- Require students to bring picture identification to the exam, if identity is a concern.

- Have students sign the cover sheet of the test.

- Instruct students not to leave their seats, but to raise their hands if they have a question.

- Never leave a student alone. Establish a bathroom policy before the test.

- Collect the test materials from students while they remain seated to avoid confusion and distraction at the front of the room.

- Look carefully at each answer sheet and test booklet as you collect them to make sure that they have accurate identifying information, and make sure that there are no stray marks on the answer sheets.

- Use an attendance sheet to carefully check that all test material is collected.

- Develop a make-up test policy that discourages students from missing a scheduled exam.

ACADEMIC INTEGRITY POLICY   What are the consequences for cheating? This is a question that troubles educators, but it is a question that must be answered. First of all, you must understand the policy of your institution. Policies and procedures regarding cheating can be found on virtually every college campus (Cizak, 1999). Make sure that you are aware of these policies and that the policy established in a nursing department is congruent with the institution's policy.

The consequences for cheating must be established and documented for both teachers and students before the semester begins. The faculty must agree on the evidence required to establish cheating and its subsequent consequences. Should two proctors agree that students are surreptitiously sharing information? Are there degrees of cheating—ranging from the student who glances across the aisle to see another answer sheet, to the student who obtains a copy of the test before the exam? What are the grading consequences? Will students be allowed to finish the test and lose credit? Or, will students who cheat receive a zero on the test? Whatever decisions are made, it is crucial that you proceed cautiously and make sure that the evidence of cheating is well documented.

The activities that define cheating and the punishment associated with that activity must be clearly communicated to the students. However, even when a cheating policy is well defined, teachers are often uneasy about accusing a student of cheating. You certainly do not want to jump to conclusions and unjustly accuse an honest student of cheating. If you detect that students are attempting to share information, or that a student is paying great attention to the answer sheet of a classmate, eye contact and extra vigilance usually discourages the activity. If it does not, quietly change their seats. It is a good policy to keep a seat or two free at the front of the room for this purpose.

If you are certain that a student or students are cheating, you are fully justified in taking the action that has been predetermined by the faculty. Ensure that you have carefully documented the event and that you save any evidence. If you have to remove a student from the classroom, try to keep the disruption to a minimum. In some situations, it may cause less disruption for the rest of the class to remove any violating materials, change the seat assignment, and allow the accused student to finish the test.

Scoring a Test

When items on a test are equally weighted, a raw score represents the number of questions that a student answered correctly. After a test is administered, it must be scored, either by hand or by machine, in order to determine the raw score. Having the students use separate answer sheets facilitates both of these scoring methods. Obviously, it is important that the students clearly understand the directions for using the answer sheet so that an accurate raw score can be determined.

If you have to score your multiple-choice exams by hand, you can create a scoring template, which is simply an answer sheet with a hole punched out for each of the correct answers. Place the template over a student's answer sheet and fill in each hole that is blank with a red mark. When you remove the template, you can count the number of red marks to determine how many questions were answered incorrectly.

An essential detail of scoring is the accuracy of the key. Whatever method you use for scoring, you must make sure that the key is correct before you start the process. First, circle the correct answers on a copy of the test and fill in the answer key based on the keyed copy of the test. Then, have two people double-check the key. One person should read the answers on the key out loud while the other checks that the key corresponds to the answers circled on the test.

With the wide availability of reasonably priced optical scanning equipment, many schools electronically score objective classroom tests. If the scanner is not interfaced with a test development program, you will have to create a key by hand. If you are using a test development software package, it will interface with the scanning hardware to score the exam. These packages eliminate the need for teacher-generated keys because the tests are scored directly from the item bank where the correct answers are stored. Most of these programs will alert you if a student has marked two answers or has omitted an answer. However, it is a good idea to examine each answer sheet for stray marks, incomplete erasures, or omitted answers before you start the scanning process. When implemented properly, electronic scoring is efficient and accurate, and can provide you with detailed analyses of the test results. These analyses offer invaluable information for translating a raw score into a meaningful inference of student achievement.

Statistical Analysis

Raw scores can be misleading. They do not always accurately reflect a student's achievement. Despite all your efforts, mistakes do occur. Errors such as miskeyed items, items having more than one correct answer, items that are too difficult for the group, or items that mislead students can creep into even the best planned exam. Thus, a teacher who simply scored a test and assigned grades without reviewing the results of the test would be very misguided.

Once you have determined the raw scores for a test, you need to analyze the results to determine the final scores. Using a computer program that provides this information is the most efficient way to approach this analysis. In fact, it is much too time-consuming for most teachers to attempt to calculate item data on their own. Teachers who do not obtain computer printouts for their exams are at an extreme disadvantage when trying to determine the accuracy of a raw score. For this reason alone, every teacher should have access to a computer analysis of their classroom tests in order to conduct a quantitative review of the test. Chapter 10, "Interpreting Test Results," examines the use of statistical analysis for quantitative review before assigning final scores to your exams.

Student Review

In addition to the faculty qualitative review before the test and the statistical review after the test, having a student qualitative review will provide you with valuable information for determining the final scores of a test, based on the opinion of the test consumers. It is best to hold a student review after the test analysis is done, but before the grades are assigned. The purpose of a test review is twofold: 1) to help students learn about their reasoning processes, and 2) to identify any undetected ambiguities in the test. Allowing students to review the exam before the grades are assigned also provides you with insight when determining what to do with a problem item.

A student review should not be a debate session, where students confront teachers to argue for more points. Nor should it simply consist of a teacher reading the correct answers to the students. Student test reviews can be productive exercises in critical thinking when students are given the opportunity to think about their thinking; to examine the process by which they chose their answers.

Because test security is a major concern, student reviews should be held in a strictly controlled setting. Many of the same restrictions, which are applied during the test, should be enforced during the review session. Students should be required to leave all pencils, pens, notes, texts, electronic devices, hats, sunglasses, and so on at the front of the room. In addition to the faculty member who is reviewing the test, proctors should also circulate to monitor the room.

It is inadvisable to give students their original answer sheets or test booklets. Many of the test development programs provide individual printouts of students' answers. If these are not available, give students photocopies of their answer sheets. A test that is developed from a software program can be projected to a wall screen from a computer, or overhead transparencies of the test can be made for projection. If students report discrepancies between the score report and their recollection of their answers on the original answer sheet, a faculty member should review the original answer sheets with the students on an individual basis.

It is preferable to hold the group review after all students have taken the exam. If students were absent on exam day, the review should be postponed until all students have taken the exam. Even if the make-up test is an alternate form, the students who have not taken the exam will have an unfair advantage if a review is held before they take the test. At the very least, students who have not taken the exam should not be allowed to attend the review.

Approach the test review as a learning experience. Start the session by telling the students that the purpose of the review is to help them improve their skills in taking multiple-choice exams that require higher order thinking. Read each question and ask students to identify the correct answer. Explain why the correct answer is correct and why the distractors are wrong. Ask for student volunteers who answered each item incorrectly to explain their thinking and discuss the inconsistencies in their logic. If students have a reasonable argument about the correctness of an option or the clarity of a stem, tell them that you will consider their input when determining the final scores. Remember not to make any promises or to take the students' comments personally. Most importantly, try to keep the atmosphere positive.

In order to avoid spending an inordinate amount of time in test review, many faculty allow students to present a written justification for an answer within a certain deadline after the test review. Haladyna (1997, p. 235) cites the following positive effects that can result from this practice:

- Encourages the students to write persuasively and think critically about their reasoning

- Recognizes when the students have a correct, creative alternative solution

- Identifies when lack of learning and/or teaching exists

- Provides an opportunity for students to vent their feelings

- Allows students to gain extra points if their justification is accepted

- Promotes a positive learning environment

If you set a deadline for submission of one to two days after the class review, you will have time to integrate the students' proposals for alternative solutions with the quantitative analysis of the test (covered in Chapter 10, "Interpreting Test Results") before you assign grades to the exam.

Many nurse educators find test review sessions to be very unpleasant. However, if you present students with a well-crafted exam that follows the guidelines presented in this book, and you give the students an opportunity to express their opinions (written or verbal), student contentiousness will be kept to a minimum. You will also find that positive review sessions and the students' written justifications will provide you with ideas for item revision. Pay attention to the students' reasoning processes and make note of their comments and ideas—they can be very helpful for item analysis as well as for future item development.

Summary

As with all aspects of the assessment process, a systematic approach to assembling, administering, and scoring multiple-choice exams decreases error and safeguards the validity and reliability of your classroom tests. These steps are often overlooked as the clerical aspects of test development, yet they are essential for the integrity of your exams. The practical guidelines offered in this chapter will help you to streamline these processes and enable you to put a professional touch on your tests.

The issues of cheating, scoring, and student test review are addressed in this chapter. Because cheating affects both the honest and dishonest students by interfering with the test's reliability, educators are responsible for taking measures to ensure the integrity of the testing environment. Strategies for detecting and interfering with student cheating are proposed to assist nursing faculty in developing a plan to ensure the integrity of test administration.

Guidelines for including student assessment through post hoc test review are also suggested. Student comments can be a valuable resource for assigning final test scores and for improving items for future use. Approaches for conducting a productive student test review are offered with a focus on the positive benefits for both students and teachers.

9 Establishing Evidence of Reliability and Validity

"Perhaps the two most important technical concepts in measurement are reliability and validity."

—William Mehrens

The two most important questions to ask about a measurement instrument are

- *How accurate is the score?*
- *How meaningful is the interpretation of the score?*

The first question challenges the instrument's reliability, while the second examines its validity.

Just how important are the concepts of reliability and validity to assessment? They are essential. They form the very basis on which fairness and trustworthiness are established. If teachers are to have confidence in the decisions they make, they must be assured that the instruments they are using are both valid and reliable.

There is an additional concern that cannot be overlooked. Students today are becoming more sophisticated. They are starting to question the reliability and validity of the assessments upon which their futures depend. In today's litigious society, it is not outside the realm of possibility that teachers could be called upon to defend their assessment decisions in a court of law. Whether it be to justify the fairness of your grade assignments or to defend yourself in a formal legal proceeding, how well prepared are you to defend your current measurement instruments?

In order to select, develop, and fairly interpret the results of measurement instruments, it is essential that you have a clear understanding of the concepts related to both reliability and validity. Reliability and validity are introduced in Chapter 2, "The Language of Assessment."

This chapter will examine how evidence of reliability and validity are established. Review of these concepts is designed to provide you with a foundation for understanding reliability and validity estimates of your classroom assessments. You will also find the information useful for selecting and interpreting the results of standardized tests.

Reliability

Reliability refers to the consistency of test results, or how constant scores are from one measurement event to another (Linn & Gronlund, 2000). Reliability is not about the test. It is about the particular sample that takes the test. In other words, it is sample-dependent. A measurement is said to be reliable if it is reproducible: If an independent replication of the same measurement on the same individual would yield the same score. A student would attain the same score on a reliable test regardless of when the test was completed, when the test was scored, or who scored the test (Moskal & Leydens, 2000). In other words, reliable tests produce trustworthy results. Chapter 2, "The Language of Assessment," discusses the various factors which influence the reliability of a test.

No test is 100 percent reliable: Error is inherent in every type of measurement. Reliability is related to the degree to which test scores are free from measurement error. The lower the error of a measurement, the more consistent test scores will be at accurately reflecting a student's actual status (Popham, 1999). While error can never be completely eliminated from an educational measurement, it is important to identify how imperfect the instrument is. Is it trustworthy enough for your purposes? Or, is it so unreliable that you cannot have confidence in the results?

Measures of Reliability

Several methods are available to help you estimate the reliability of your test scores. Because of measurement error, we can expect a certain amount of variation from one testing episode to another. Although we cannot expect our test scores to be perfect, there should be a limit to the amount of error we are willing to tolerate (Frisbe, 1988). Reliability measures provide an estimate of the consistency of the test score. There are three different approaches for obtaining evidence about reliability—test-retest, parallel-form, and internal consistency. A reliability coefficient obtained from one of these approaches is not interchangeable with a value derived by a different technique. These values are not equivalent because each incorporates a unique definition of measurement error (AERA, et al., 1999).

TEST-RETEST   One method for determining a test's reliability is to collect evidence about its stability by giving the identical test to the same individuals on a second occasion and then determining the correlation between the two sets of scores (Anastasi & Urbina, 1997). The time interval between the two administrations can vary from a few days to several years. Longer time periods between testing will result in lower reliability because of changes in the students. Therefore, it is important to note the time interval when reporting test-retest reliability. The major drawback of this approach is that it requires that the exact same test be given to the same individuals on two different occasions, a situation that is usually not feasible in a classroom situation.

PARALLEL-FORM RELIABILITY   Parallel-form reliability evidence is concerned with the comparability of two alternate forms of a test. With this method the same person is tested with two different forms of a test. The reliability of the test is represented by the correlation of the scores on the two forms of the test (Anastasi & Urbina, 1997). Because of the difficulty in constructing two equivalent forms of the same test, this method is not a likely alternative for most classroom teachers. In addition, students most likely would object to duplicate testing for the sake of obtaining reliability. If the parallel forms are administered at different times, then the time interval between testing episodes must be taken into consideration when interpreting the reliability coefficient. The shorter the time interval, the higher the reliability coefficient will be.

INTERNAL CONSISTENCY   Because it is usually not practical or appropriate to repeat a classroom test, or to develop an alternative form of the test to determine its reliability, various statistical methods have been developed to estimate the reliability of a test from a single administration. These methods of analysis estimate the internal consistency of a test and report a reliability coefficient, or an index of the amount of error, for a particular test. Of the three methods for estimating reliablily, methods of internal analysis are most appropriate for use with classroom tests. These analyses can detect the errors that are most commonly associated with teacher-made tests (Frisbe, 1988).

While correlations for test-retest and parallel-form reliability tell us what we can reasonably estimate as the degree of relationship between two test scores, reliability coefficients give an estimate of internal consistency, or the degree to which the items in one test are measuring a common characteristic of a person (Thorndike, 1997). While a correlation coefficient ranges between –1.0 and +1.0, with –1.0 and +1.0 indicating perfect correlation, a reliability coefficient falls between 0.0 and 1.0. A reliability coefficient of 1.0 indicates perfect reliability, while a reliability coefficient of 0.0 indicates that the test completely lacks reliability (see Figure 9.1).

Range 0.0 to +1.0

+1.0 = PERFECT

0.0 = No Reliability

FIGURE 9.1   Reliability coefficient

There are several procedures for obtaining a reliability estimate from a single form of a test. The procedures that are most frequently reported in today's test analysis computer programs determine the reliability of the test based on the internal consistency of the test. Their formulas are based on the concept that each item in a test can be considered a one-item test (Thorndike, 1997). Internal estimates of reliability compare each item in the test to the total score on the test and depend on the variance of the test, the variance of the individual items, and the consistency of the performance of the test-takers from item to item (Thorndike, 1997). The higher the variance, or spread of scores on the test, the higher the reliability of the test.

Fortunately, you no longer have to be a computational wizard to obtain and interpret test data. With the availability of today's optical scanners and computer hardware and software, valuable test statistics are readily available to the classroom teacher. So, you have easy access to the instruments that can help you to efficiently evaluate and improve the quality of your tests. Advanced mathematical skills are not required to use this information.

Although you will not have to actually calculate test statistics, you need to be aware of the factors that influence reliability in order to facilitate your ability to interpret test results and improve your classroom assessment instruments. A logical and practical approach for interpreting statistical analysis to improve your tests and to increase your confidence in the judgments you make based on your tests is presented in Chapter 10, "Interpreting Test Results."

Just as students have different learning styles, so do faculty. I have included several formulas throughout the book for those of you who find the mathematical explanation of statistical analysis helpful. Do not let the complexity of these mathematical formulas baffle you. Only those who are involved in the psychometric analysis of test data need to have a thorough understanding of the calculations involved. Ignore them if you find them confusing; you will never need to perform any of these calculations. However, for many of you, visualizing how the factors associated with reliability affect statistical outcomes will help to demystify the calculations and diminish the intimidating nature of test data analysis.

What is important is that you understand the principles of assessment. The purpose of this discussion is to explain these principles and improve the reliability of the information you obtain from classroom tests. If you are interested in learning more about calculating reliability coefficients and other statistical test data, a clear and comprehensive presentation is provided in *Psychological Testing* (Anastasi & Urbina, 1997).

Reports of reliability calculated from internal consistency include the *split-half method*, the *Kuder-Richardson formula 20 (KR-20)*, and *coefficient alpha*. Each of these methods estimates reliability from a single form of a test.

Split-Half Reliability Coefficient   A split-half procedure arbitrarily splits the test into reasonably equivalent halves so that each individual receives two scores. These two scores are correlated and a reliability coefficient is determined. This approach yields a correlation coefficient similar to the test-retest and parallel-form methods, however, only one test is administered. This type of reliability coefficient is referred to as a measure of internal consistency because only one test is administered (Anastasi & Urbina, 1997).

The first problem that is encountered when determining split-half reliability is to decide how to split the test so that the two most equivalent halves are identified. The procedure most often used is to assign the odd-numbered questions to one half-test and the even-numbered questions to the other half-test (Thorndike, 1997). Two problems are associated with this method of estimating reliability. The first is that different estimates will result from different subdivisions of the test. Secondly, the correlation only estimates the reliability of half a test (Anastasi & Urbina, 1997). However, the second problem can be corrected by using the Spearman-Brown prophecy formula which adjusts the correlation to estimate the reliability of the whole test (Nitko, 1996).

Kuder-Richardson (KR-20) and Coefficient Alpha Reliability Coefficients
While the split-half reliability is derived from a planned split of a test, the reliability coefficients derived from the coefficient alpha and the KR-20 formulas are actually the

average of all the split-half coefficients that can be derived from all possible splittings of a test (Anastasi & Urbina, 1997). Estimates provided by these formulas are really indications of the degree to which the individual item responses correlate with the total test score, or how well a test correlates with itself (Mehrens & Lehmann, 1973). Both of these estimates of reliability provide information about the degree to which the test items are measuring similar characteristics (Linn & Gronlund, 2000).

$$KR_{20} = \frac{N}{N-1} \times \frac{SD_t^2 - \Sigma PQ}{SD_t^2}$$

N = Number of items on the test

SD_t^2 = Variance of the test scores

Σ = Sum of

P = Proportion answering an item correctly

Q = Proportion answering an item incorrectly

FIGURE 9.2   Kuder-Richardson formula

$$\alpha = \frac{N}{N-1} \times \frac{SD_t^2 - \Sigma SD_i^2}{SD_t^2}$$

N = Number of items on the test

α = Coefficient alpha

SD_t^2 = Variance of the test scores

Σ = Sum of

SD_i^2 = Variance of the individual items on the test

FIGURE 9.3   Coefficient alpha

The KR-20 formula, shown in Figure 9.2, is used when each item on a test is scored dichotomously, that is, either correct or incorrect. When the items are not scored dichotomously, the formula for coefficient alpha, shown in Figure 9.3, is used. The two formulas are essentially the same, except that in coefficient alpha, ΣPQ is replaced by ΣSD_i^2, which is the sum of all the item variances (Anastasi & Urbina, 1997, p. 98). Coefficient alpha is the only commonly available computer-calculated reliability estimate for instruments whose items can take on a range of values, such as in a personality inventory (Worthen, Borg, & White, 1993, p. 157). It can actually be used to measure reliability for instruments with either dichotomous or weighted scores (because the ΣSD_i^2 is equal to ΣPQ).

The KR-20 and coefficient alpha estimates are most frequently used by test publishers and are reported by most classroom test development software packages. They provide an estimate of the reliability for the total test score based on the consistency with which students respond from one item on a test to the next. Examine the formulas for both the KR-20 and the coefficient alpha (Figures 9.2 and 9.3). They clarify that the higher the variance (SD^2), the higher the reliablility of the test. This means that the more scores on a test are spread out from the mean, the higher the test reliability.

Measurement Error

Measurement error decreases the usefulness of a test. Previous discussion has established that no measurement is perfect; they all contain error. Some kinds of physical measurement, such as weight and height, have been perfected to the point that, with a good measurement procedure, error is relatively small. In contrast, measurements of behavior contain a larger margin of error. Although we cannot expect tests to provide perfect measurements, there is a limit to how much error we should accept. The greater the confidence that you require when interpreting a test score, the lower the error and the higher the reliability you must require of a test.

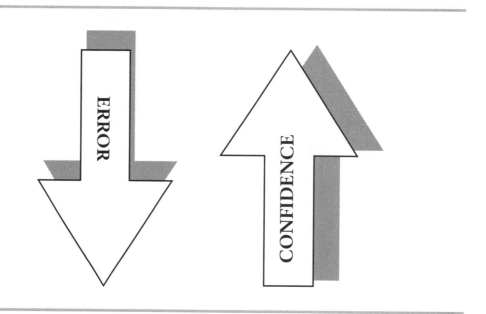

FIGURE 9.4   Lower error results in higher score confidence

STANDARD ERROR OF MEASUREMENT (SEM)   While the reliability estimates that we have examined so far are concerned with the reliability of test scores for a group, the standard error of measurement (SEM) is concerned with the consistency with which we measure an individual's performance (Popham, 1999). An individual's true score is one that is free from error and can be obtained only if a test is perfectly reliable. As we know, perfect reliability is not attainable; error is inherent in every measurement. Although we cannot eliminate measurement error, we can estimate how much error is present in an instrument. This estimation is the SEM: The smaller the SEM, the more reliable the test score.

Although we can never know what an individual's true score is, we can estimate the amount by which an obtained score may differ from the hypothetical true score. If we were able to repeatedly administer the same test to an individual, we would see that the person's scores would vary somewhat from one administration to another and the distribution of these obtained scores would be normal in shape. The individual's hypothetical true test score would be equal to the average score of this normal distribution of obtained scores and the SEM would be equal to the standard deviation of the distribution (Lyman, 1998).

The SEM reflects the consistency of an individual's scores if the same test were given to that student over and over again. The amount of variation in the scores from one administration to the next would be directly related to the reliability of the test. The higher the reliability of the test, the less the individual's score would vary from one administration to another (Linn & Gronlund, 2000). Because it is not possible to repeatedly reassess a student, an estimation of an individual's true score is derived from a mathematical equation that combines information about the reliability coefficient and the standard deviation of the test (Worthen, Borg, & White, 1993, p. 118). As the formula in Figure 9.5 illustrates, the higher the reliability of a test and the smaller the standard deviation, the lower the SEM.

$$SEM = SD \sqrt{1 - r^n}$$

SD = Standard deviation

r^n = Reliability coefficient of the test

FIGURE 9.5   Standard error of measurement (SEM) formula

CONFIDENCE BANDS   The SEM, which is reported as score units, is particularly useful because it is directly applicable to test score interpretations. It provides us with a safeguard against placing too much emphasis on a single score (Anastasi & Urbina, 1997, p. 109). The SEM tells us how many points should be added to and subtracted from an individual's score to estimate the "reasonable limits" in which the true score most probably can be found. These reasonable limits provide a confidence band for estimating an individual's true score (Linn & Gronlund, 2000).

The SEM reminds us of the imprecision of a single test score. The score report in Table 9.1 shows that a student has a math score of 500 with an SEM of 10. The SEM of 10 allows us to estimate that this student's true score is likely to be in the range that is 10 points above or below the student's obtained score of 500. Note that the student has obtained the same verbal score of 500. However, this score has a much larger SEM (50) which means that the student's true verbal score lies somewhere in the range of 450 to 550, a much larger confidence band.

While we cannot eliminate measurement error, the goal of test construction is to decrease measurement error and increase reliability. As error decreases, confidence increases. A large confidence band indicates large measurement error and decreases the confidence that we can have in the obtained score. With low error, the confidence band decreases and we can be more confident that the obtained score is a dependable measure. As Table 9.1 illustrates, we can have more confidence in an obtained score of

TABLE 9.1   Score report with score range illustrating confidence band

	Score	SEM	Score Range
Math	500	10	490–510
Verbal	500	50	450–550

500 with a score range of 490 to 510 than we can in an obtained score of 500 with a score range of 450 to 550. The message for teachers is clear: Because of measurement error, you must interpret a student's obtained score as an estimate of the true score (Nitko, 1996).

Because the SEM represents the standard deviation of the hypothetical distribution around a student's true score, the SEM can be interpreted in terms of the normal curve (McMillan, 1997, p. 362). In a normal curve, approximately 68 percent of the cases fall within one standard deviation of the mean, approximately 95 percent of the scores will fall between the mean and two standard deviations, and nearly all of the scores, greater than 99 percent, will fall within three standard deviations from the mean (Anastasi & Urbina, 1997, p. 54).

How should we interpret the obtained score for our student who has a math score of 500 with an SEM of 10? As Table 9.2 illustrates, a confidence band of one standard error above and one standard error below the obtained score would allow us 68 percent confidence that the student's true score falls between 490 and 510; a confidence band of two standard errors above and two standard errors below the obtained score would allow us 95 percent confidence that the student's true score falls between 480 and 520; and a confidence band of three standard errors above and three standard errors below the obtained score would allow us greater than 99 percent confidence that the student's true score falls between 470 and 530 (McMillan, 1997, p.362). Compare Table 9.2 to Table 9.3.

TABLE 9.2   Degree of Confidence Associated with SEM

MATH SCORE = 500   SEM = 10

Degree of Confidence	Number of Standard Errors	Range of Scores or Confidence Band
68%	1	490–510
95%	2	480–520
99.7%	3	470–530

Although the student has the same obtained score for both math and verbal, the difference in their SEMs results in much different confidence bands, further illustrating that the smaller the confidence band, the greater confidence you can have in an obtained score. Consider that with three standard errors of measurement the student's true verbal score would be in the range of 350 to 650! Although we can be 99 percent confident that the student's true score falls within this interval, with such a large interval it is difficult to have much confidence in the student's obtained verbal score.

TABLE 9.3 Degree of Confidence Associated with Large SEM

VERBAL SCORE = 500   SEM = 50

Degree of Confidence	Number of Standard Errors	Range of Scores or Confidence Band
68%	1	450–550
95%	2	400–600
99.7%	3	350–650

If we interpret a person's obtained score as equivalent to the true score we will make serious misinterpretations. It is important to interpret a student's obtained score in relation to a confidence band, and to remember that we do not know where on the interval the student's true score lies. The most accurate way to interpret a student's score is to view it in terms of an interval, not as a single score.

Professionally developed standardized tests are subject to measurement error. Therefore, it is reasonable to assume that classroom tests also contain measurement error. This error makes it impossible to be dogmatic when interpreting test results, and clearly illustrates that assigning grades in a course should never be based on the results of one measurement. It is important to collect as much information as possible and consider measurement error when making assessment decisions about students based on classroom assessments.

Validity

If a test is to be useful, it must be reliable; but reliability alone is not enough. The interpretations that you make of a test's results must have evidence of validity. Validity is the most important aspect of a test; it refers to the degree to which evidence supports your interpretations of the test, not to the test itself.

Classroom tests are designed so that teachers can make decisions about a student's achievement. High scores lead to one type of inference, while low scores lead to the opposite conclusion. These test-based inferences may or may not be valid. It is the validity of the inferences made based on classroom assessments with which teachers must be concerned when making decisions about students. If the inferences are accurate, then the resulting decisions are defensible (Popham, 1999, p. 42).

The *Standards for Educational and Psychological Testing* states that, "Validity is a unitary concept. It is the degree to which all the accumulated evidence supports the intended interpretation of test scores for the proposed purpose" (AERA, et al., 1999, p. 11). If a test is interpreted in more than one way, each interpretation must be validated. Refer to Chapter 2, "The Language of Assessment," to review the discussion of the unitary nature of validity and the three types of evidence that support the validity of the interpretations of a measurement instrument—content-related, construct-related, and criterion-related.

Content Validity Index

While there are no objective empirical methods for obtaining content-related evidence of validity, it is possible to use interrater agreement indexes, such as the content validity index (CVI), to rate the relevance of the items on a measurement instrument. With this procedure, a panel of experts is asked to rate the content relevance of each item on a scale of 1 to 4 (Burns & Grove, 1997; Lynn, 1986; Polit & Hungler, 1999). The CVI for the total instrument is the percentage of total items that are rated by the experts as 3 or 4. Polit and Hungler suggest that a CVI of 0.80 or better indicates good measurement reliability. If this procedure were to be used to rate the items on a multiple-choice exam, it would have to be used during the test development process, and then only items that were rated as highly relevant to the blueprint should be included in the test.

Determining the CVI would involve a time commitment that precludes its effectiveness for classroom exams. A group of faculty, who were expert in the field but not involved in developing the blueprint or test items, would have to serve as the panel of experts to rate each item for relevance to the individual test blueprint and to identify areas of omission before the test is administered. However, considering the rigorous nature of the process and the number of exams that are administered each semester, it would not be feasible to carry out this procedure for every classroom exam.

The most important requirement for establishing content-related evidence of validity for a classroom exam is to follow the guidelines presented in this book to build in validity from the beginning of test development. While it may be helpful to determine the CVI on a few selected exams, be careful not to be misled. Numbers in themselves do not lend credence to evidence of validity. The most effective and practical approach for content validation of a classroom achievement test is to develop and select items according to a carefully designed test blueprint.

Interpretation of the Validity Coefficient

Test developers frequently establish criterion-related and construct-related evidence of validity by calculating correlation coefficients to measure the relationship between the test and the criterion. While there is no objective numerical value associated with evidence of content-related validity, criterion-related and construct-related evidence can be reported as a validity coefficient. A validity coefficient is a correlation coefficient that expresses the relationship between two sets of scores.

The Pearson product-moment correlation coefficient is the most common procedure used for reporting validity. A number ranging between –1 and +1 represents the direction and strength of the relationship between two sets of continuous scores. The direction of the relationship is indicated by the positive or negative value and the strength of the relationship is indicated by the numerical value from –1 to 0 or from 0 to +1 (McMillan, 1997).

A correlation coefficient (r) of +1 indicates a perfect positive correlation between the predictor and the criterion, while r = –1 indicates a perfect negative correlation. The closer a validity coefficient is to +1, the more accurate the test at predicting the criterion. For example, a validity coefficient of 0.95 applied to the relationship between the scores on a nursing school entrance exam and first year grade point average is a high positive relationship and the test would have considerable predictive ability. However, because all measurements contain error, caution must be taken when interpreting correlations. Test scores should be interpreted as a range when estimating current performance or predicting future performance on a criterion (McMillan, 1997).

While classroom teachers seldom conduct formal studies to obtain correlation coefficients, the concept is important to understand. As McMillan explains, "when you have two or more measures of the same thing, and these measures provide similar results, then you have established, albeit informally, criterion-related evidence" (1997, p. 58). For example, if your assessment of a student's critical thinking ability in clinical practice coincides with the student's score on a test that measures critical thinking ability, then you have criterion-related evidence that your inference about the student's critical thinking ability is valid. This reasoning gives further support to the notion that it is important to obtain several measurements of the same constructs and content in order to support the validity of your interpretations.

Summary

Reliability is concerned with the consistency of test results. Sound decisions cannot be based on a test that produces inconsistent results. The higher the stakes associated with the use of a test, the more concerned we have to be with the test's reliability.

The three types of evidence about a test's consistency are: test-retest, parallel-form, and internal consistency. Although these three kinds of evidence are related, they are not interchangeable. While test-retest and parallel-form evidence of reliability provide correlations between sets of student scores, internal consistency is concerned with the extent to which the test's items are functioning in a consistent fashion (Popham, 1999). The measurements produced by these different approaches are not equivalent or interchangeable.

The intended use of test scores affects the type of reliability evidence that is required. Classroom tests are most amenable to internal consistency measures. In all cases, when we are concerned with interpreting the score of an individual, the standard error of measurement is the best index of consistency.

Validity is the most important aspect of test development. "A sound validity argument integrates various strands of evidence into a coherent account of the degree to which existing evidence and theory support the intended interpretation of test scores for specific uses" (AERA, et al., 1999, p. 17). Establishing evidence of validity must begin during the test development process in order to justify that the selected set of items represents the domain being measured.

Reliability and validity form the basis for all assessment. A test that is valid and reliable measures what it intends to measure with a degree of accuracy that can be trusted. Considering the serious decisions that are made about students based on classroom tests, faculty should have a working knowledge of the concepts of reliability and validity. An understanding of these concepts will provide you with a framework both for developing more effective tests and for accurately interpreting and using test results. It will also enable you to design methods to collect the evidence of validity and reliability that you will need to document when you seek program accreditation.

10 Interpreting Test Results

"Accept the fact that regardless of how many times you are right, you will sometimes be wrong."

—Jackson H. Brown

Test development is a process that continues even after a test is administered. In fact, post-hoc test analysis is a crucial aspect of the process. If you neglect to review an exam after it is scored, it is likely that you will be making decisions based on inaccurate test results. Test analysis has three goals: to identify whether any of the questions are flawed, to correct any errors and adjust the raw scores, and to improve the items for future use. As Gullickson and Ellwein (1985) point out, measurement experts agree that post-hoc statistical analysis of a test is an essential testing tool. Without statistical analysis, you cannot have assurance that your tests are functioning as you intended.

Qualitative and quantitative test reviews are equally important; they complement each other. Once you have the statistical data for a test, you will be able to look at the items from a much more objective viewpoint. Inevitably, you and your colleagues who reviewed the exam before it was administered will be surprised by the results of at least ten percent of the new items on a test even though you carefully followed test development guidelines. Sometimes, student responses to even the most expertly written questions are just unpredictable.

Consider the time invested in item writing and revision as an investment. Multiple-choice items can be analyzed, revised, and "banked" for future use. These items can be polished over time and adapted for use and reused for years to come. Often the qualitative student review, as discussed in Chapter 8, "Assembling, Administering, and Scoring a Test," will explain the statistical results of an item and will provide suggestions for revising the items for future use.

Reviewing the quantitative data not only provides you with an invaluable tool for making objective decisions about individual test items and overall test scores, but it also guides you so that you use your time efficiently to improve your questions and develop a valuable testing resource: an item bank. Keep in mind that the more items you analyze, the more proficient you become at writing and identifying high-quality test items that you can bank and use repeatedly. Therefore, the time you invest is time well spent.

Before the advent of reasonably priced testing software, calculating the statistical results of an exam was a task that was impractical for a classroom teacher. Today, many colleges and universities provide machine scoring with statistical reports of test and item analysis for multiple-choice classroom exams. The aim of this chapter is to demonstrate just how valuable this data is as a tool for test interpretation and development. The ultimate goal is to convince you to take full advantage of this service if your institution provides it or to lobby your administration to provide this service if it does not currently do so.

Overall Test Data Analysis

Most test development software packages provide two levels of test analysis data. The first is the overall analysis of the test, and the second is a detailed analysis of each item as it relates to the test as a whole. While your first consideration should be to look at the overall picture, both of these data sets are essential for a thorough test analysis. Examining test data is well within your purview once you understand the meaning of each of the values. Remember, you do not have to do any actual calculating. Once you use the data, you will appreciate its value to such an extent that I guarantee you will never again assign grades to a multiple-choice exam without reviewing the statistical analysis.

When a test is scored, the initial result is reported as a raw score or the number of items that a student answered correctly on the test. Statistical analysis assists you with transforming the raw scores into test grades. Appendix A, "Basic Test Statistics," defines basic test statistics. Take the time to review those definitions before examining the example of a statistical test report in Table 10.1.

TABLE 10.1   Sample Test Statistics

Number of Items	100
Number of Examinees	92
Mean	75.4
Median	77
Low Score	52
High Score	93
Alpha	0.754
Standard Deviation	7.7
SEM	3.8
Mean p-value	0.7540
Mean PBI	0.36

Table 10.1 is a sample test analysis report that contains the typical data that you would receive from a testing software program. In fact, this report presents more than enough data to help you make informed decisions about test results. Some programs provide even more comprehensive statistics. It is not necessary to make your review too complicated, however; this sample data is more than sufficient for analysis of a classroom test.

Generally, item statistics for small groups of students will be relatively unstable. The stability of test analysis data increases as the number of students approaches 100. Therefore, when you have a very small group (50 or fewer), you must consider the relative instability of the data when you interpret the analysis. In fact, test and item analysis should not be interpreted dogmatically, no matter how large the number of students. As this discussion will illustrate, analysis of test data requires a variety of interpretations, both qualitative and quantitative. The size of the sample is one of the factors that you must consider.

The first step in test analysis is to review the report to make sure that the data is complete. Check the number of items and examinees and verify that they are accurate. This sample has 100 items, which means that the raw score is equal to the percent correct, and 92 examinees had their answer sheets scored. Once you verify that these figures are correct, you are ready to analyze the results of the test.

Measures of Central Tendency

Measures of central tendency provide a single value that best represents the typical score in a distribution. The mean, the median, and the mode are the three measures that are the most commonly used measures of central tendency in education. While the mode, which represents the most frequently obtained score in a distribution, has limited usefulness for interpreting classroom test scores, both the mean and the median provide valuable information.

MEAN   Most test analysis programs report the mean, or arithmetic average, of the raw scores on the test. In this case it is 75.4. The mean percent score is determined by dividing the mean raw score by the total number of items on the test. The mean percent score is equal to the mean raw score in this example because there are 100 items on the test. It is important to examine the relationship of the mean to the passing standard that you have set. If, for example, your passing standard is 75 percent, this test has an average score at the passing level. Several factors must be considered when interpreting the mean:

- What was the quality of teaching on a range between effective and ineffective?

- What was the students' level of effort to achieve the outcomes on a range between maximal and minimal?

- Where did the material/objectives fit on a range between too easy and too difficult?

- How difficult were the items on a range between too easy and too hard?

If a test has a very low mean, you should be alerted to investigate whether there is a problem with one of these factors. As Haladyna (1997) points out, if you intentionally give difficult tests, you should adjust your grading policy to ensure that you assign grades fairly in relation to the other courses that the students take. Similar consideration should be made if your tests are consistently too easy. The ideal goal is to have a test with a mean that reflects a range of student abilities. A test should be neither too easy nor too difficult but should reward those students who are high achievers and should identify those who have not met the course objectives. Chapter 11, "Assigning Grades," discusses the issues surrounding grade assignment.

MEDIAN

The median in this sample is 77, which represents the middle point in this group of raw scores. In a normal distribution, the mean and the median are the same. If a distribution is positively skewed, meaning that the test is very difficult for the group with a majority of the scores at the low end of the distribution and few very high scores, the mean will be pulled to the positive end of the distribution and will be higher than the median (Worthen, Borg, & White, 1993, p. 101).

A positively skewed distribution, such as the one depicted in Figure 10.1 signals a problem. Why are there so few high scores? What went wrong in the instructional process?

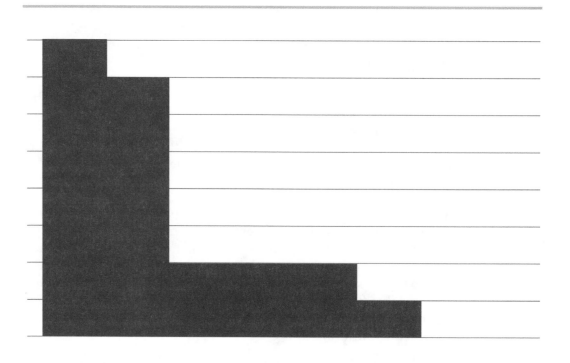

FIGURE 10.1   A positively skewed distribution

If a distribution is negatively skewed, it means that the test was easy for the group with a majority of the scores at the high end of the distribution and few very low scores. The distribution that is depicted in Figure 10.2 is one that you might expect in a nursing class. After all, all of the students are capable of successfully achieving the objectives. You cannot make assumptions about a test without examining all of the analysis data, however.

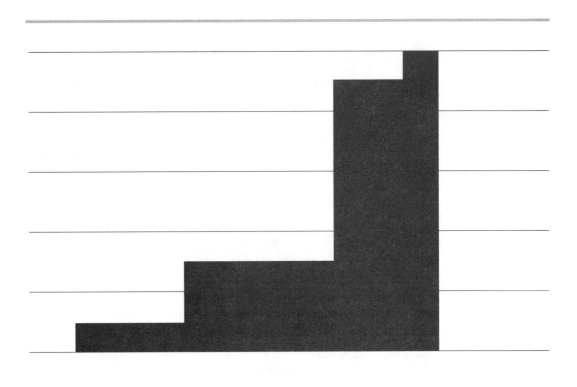

FIGURE 10.2 A negatively skewed distribution

The mean in a negatively skewed distribution is pulled toward the negative end of the distribution and will be lower than the median (Worthen, Borg, & White, 1993, p. 101). Therefore, the mean can give the wrong impression whenever a distribution is seriously skewed. In those cases, it is best to use the median as the best representation of a set of scores (Lyman, 1998). The mean and median in the example of Table 10.1 are close, which means that there are probably not many extreme scores in the distribution and the mean can be interpreted as representing a typical score, or the central tendency of the test. Of course, you will need to review the score distribution, which is also included in the test analysis report, before you decide whether the mean actually represents a typical score. Frequency and graphic distributions interpretation are discussed later in this chapter.

Measures of Variability

Because it is impossible to predict the range of scores for a test based on measures of central tendency alone, it is necessary for us to look further when interpreting a set of scores. In fact, two sets of scores could have the same mean and have a very different spread of scores. We need to examine measures of variability to determine how much the scores spread out from the mean or how much dispersion there is in a distribution.

RANGE   In the example in Table 10.1, the range of the distribution is 41, the difference between the high (93) and low (52) scores on the test. A small range indicates a concentrated distribution of scores. A large range means that the scores are spread out and that some students have not done well on the test. This value gives us a rough idea of the variability of the test scores. The standard deviation is a much better measure of variability of a score distribution, however.

STANDARD DEVIATION (SD)   The standard deviation (in our example, 7.665) is the most dependable measure of variability (Lyman, 1998). As Chapter 9, "Establishing Evidence of Reliability and Validity," discusses, a large variance indicates that the scores are spread out from the mean. Conversely, the smaller the variance, the greater the similarity of the scores and the closer they are to the mean. Most software programs report the standard deviation, which is the square root of the variance, in their test analyses reports. The standard deviation is most useful for making interpretations about the normal curve, which is a grading method that is discouraged for classroom testing as Chapter 11, "Assigning Grades," discusses. In the classroom setting, the most useful application of the standard deviation is to help you to understand the reliability and standard error of measurement (SEM) for a test.

Reliability Coefficient

As Chapter 2, "The Language of Assessment," and Chapter 9, "Establishing Evidence of Reliability and Validity," discuss at length, reliability refers to the amount of confidence you can have in a set of test scores. The reliability for our sample in Table 10.1 is reported as alpha, and its value is 0.754.

What reliability should you expect from your classroom exams? The answer to this question varies, but it relates directly to the level of confidence that you must have in the decisions that are made based on the test results. High-stakes decisions require measurements with high reliability. In other words, a test that decides whether a student will graduate would require a high level of reliability. For this reason, you should never base such a serious decision on just one classroom exam—particularly one that has low reliability.

Linn and Gronlund (2000) agree that the degree of reliability you must require for a classroom test depends largely on the decision to be made based on the test. Consider the importance of the decision and whether the decision can be reversed. If the reliability of a test is low, make sure that you make tentative decisions, obtain additional data, and, most importantly, are willing to reverse your decision.

Linn and Gronlund (2000) report that the reliability of teacher-made tests usually varies between 0.60 and 0.85. Kehoe (1995) maintains that tests of more than 50 items should have reliability coefficients of greater than 0.80. Frisbe (1988) asserts that teacher-made tests tend to yield reliability coefficients that average about 0.50 and that 0.85 is the generally acceptable minimum reliability standard when decisions are being made about individuals based on a single score. Frisbe also states that reliabilities of about 0.50 for teacher-made tests can be tolerated when the scores will be combined with other scores to assign a grade. In that case, it is the reliability of the score that results from combining the scores with which you should be concerned.

Our sample's reliability of 0.754 looks respectable at first glance according to these standards. This value should not be considered in isolation, however. The factors that affect the reliability of a test must be taken into account. These factors are discussed in Chapter 2, "The Language of Assessment," and include the following:

- Quality of the test items

- Item difficulty

- Item discrimination

- Homogeneity of the test content

- Homogeneity of the test group

- Test length

- Number of examinees

- Speed

- Test design, administration, and scoring

When reviewing the reliability of your classroom tests, consider all of these factors. If you have a class that consists of a homogeneous group of high-achieving students, you might get a low reliability coefficient on a test of difficult, well-written, heterogeneous items that follow all of the guidelines outlined in this book. It is also possible that a low reliability indicates that the items are either too difficult or too easy for the group of students. On the other hand, you could obtain a high reliability coefficient for a speeded test with a large number of items on narrowly defined content that is administered to a large, heterogeneous group of students. Also remember that the testing conditions, quality of teaching, and number of questions and/or examinees are all factors that can affect the reliability of test scores. Low reliability coefficients are most often due to an excess of very easy or very hard items, poorly written items that do not discriminate, or test items that do not represent a unified body of content (Kehoe, 1995).

You must consider all of the influencing factors when interpreting a reliability coefficient for a test. Your judgment is a very important part of the equation. As Mark Twain said, "There are three kinds of lies: lies, damned lies, and statistics." Statistical findings are meaningless in themselves, and they can be distorted to fit erroneous interpretations. It is your informed interpretation of the data that adds the ingredient of fairness to your grade assignments.

Standard Error of Measurement (SEM)

The SEM enables us to estimate the amount by which a student's obtained score might differ from the student's true score. The SEM is very important, because if we assume that an obtained score on a test is necessarily the student's true score, we will misinterpret the test results (Lyman, 1998). The SEM for our sample is 3.8, which means that the true score for an observed raw score of 72 would range between 68.2 and 75.8. Suppose that the passing score was predetermined to be 75. Would you consider adding four points to all of the scores on the test?

It is not advisable to add points, or scale grades, for each individual test. If you are inclined to scale the grades, it is a better practice to wait for the final grade. Suppose you scale up the grades three points for exam one and the scores on exam two are very high. Will you "scale down" the scores for exam two? You probably would cause a student revolt.

Scaling individual test scores can alter the predetermined weighting of the components of the course grade (refer to Chapter 11, "Assigning Grades"). The better practice is to wait until the end of the course, look carefully at the means, reliability coefficients, and SEMs for all of the exams, consider the final score spread, and then add points (if you judge it necessary) to the final grade assignment (refer to the discussion on grading in Chapter 11).

The important lesson to be learned from the SEM is that classroom test scores are not absolute, and they do not represent students' true scores. Therefore, you must look at the margin of error in a test and be flexible when translating raw scores into test scores and test scores into course grades. If the statistical analysis provided by your test development software does not provide the SEM, you can easily calculate it by using the formula in Figure 9.5.

Mean p-value

The p-value of an item is the percent of correct responses to the item. The mean p-value identifies the average p-value of the items on a test and tells you how difficult the total test is. The mean p-value of a test translates easily into the mean percent correct score on the test (75.4 percent in the case of our sample). It is easy to see that the difficulty of the individual items is what determines the difficulty of the overall test.

Developing an item bank will help you control the difficulty of future exams. Each item should be carefully examined and revised based on the data provided before it is entered into a bank. When you store items with their data, you will have an indication of how difficult the items are when you select them for use on future tests. Remember, the difficulty of an item pertains to its use on a specific exam; it could perform differently in another item set or with a different group of students. You can get a pretty good idea of how an item will work from its history, however.

Your ability to write items at particular difficulty levels improves as you develop expertise in item writing. In addition, the more items you analyze, the more proficient you become at recognizing good items and adapting your personal style to write effective test questions. Item analysis is examined in depth later in this chapter.

It is important to note that an item's difficulty level is directly related to its ability to discriminate. If the items on a test are too easy (for example, if the average p-value is 100 percent), there will be no discrimination between the high and low scorers because everyone will have answered every item correctly. According to Kehoe (1995), a good test contains items with p-values between 0.30 and 0.80; items that are answered correctly or incorrectly by more than 85 percent of the examinees will have poor discrimination power.

How difficult should a classroom test be? Nursing faculty frequently ask this question. The reason why there is no standard response to this important question is because the answer is a very individual one. Several factors must be considered. A test is only as hard or as easy as the teacher makes it. First, you have to look at what the passing score is for the course. In many nursing programs, a grade of C is the minimum passing score. In fact, most institutions require that students maintain a grade of C or better in their major. Because C is considered "average," you must decide what "average" is in relation to your course objectives. Keeping the p-value of your items in the average range of 0.70 to 0.80, for example, will yield a test with a mean in the range between 0.70 and 0.80. At the same time, you might want to include some "easy" items (p-value above 0.80) in order to encourage students at the beginning of a test or to test important course content, and you should include some "difficult" items (p-value below 0.70) that are challenging and that identify the high-achieving students (Frary, 1995). Frary recommends limiting the number of items that more than 90 percent of the students answer correctly because these items do not contribute to the reliability of a test.

As long as the items relate to the blueprint, having a range of difficulty levels for test items will increase the variability of your test scores. Remember, the higher the score variability, the higher the test reliability.

Mean Biserial

The point biserial index (PBI) represents the discrimination ability of an item, which is the basic measure of item quality for multiple-choice tests (Kehoe, 1995). It identifies the capability of an item to distinguish between those who scored at the high end on the test and those who scored at the low end. The PBI ranges from –1.0 to +1.0; the higher the PBI, the better the item discriminates between the high and low achievers on the test. A positive PBI for an item indicates that students who achieved high scores on the test chose the correct answer for that item more frequently than students who had low scores. If students who achieved low scores on the test chose the correct answer for an item more frequently than students who have high scores, the item will have a negative biserial. When there is little or no difference between the proportion of high-scoring and low-scoring students who select the correct answer, the item contributes nothing to the reliability of the test because it does not discriminate. As Chapter 2, "The Language of Assessment," explains, the higher the average item discrimination ability, the higher the reliability of the test (Ebel, 1979, p. 268).

Just as the mean p-value represents the average difficulty of the items on the test, the mean biserial represents the average discrimination power of the items on the test. A high mean biserial indicates that the test contains high-quality items (that the items on the test discriminated between the high and low achievers). Table 10.2 summarizes Ebel's (1979, p. 267) proposed range for evaluating discrimination indices for items on classroom tests.

TABLE 10.2   Ebel's Range for Discrimination Indices

- > 0.40   Very good

- 0.30 to 0.39   Reasonably good, consider improving

- 0.20 to 0.29   Marginal, needs improvement

- < 0.19   Poor, reject or revise

Haladyna (1997, p. 240) defines a highly discriminating item on a classroom exam as one that has a PBI above 0.20 and a p-value between 0.60 and 0.90. Kehoe (1995) maintains that items that have a PBI of less than 0.15 should be restructured. The mean biserial for our sample is 0.36. According to these criteria, our sample is well within the reasonably good category. For the purposes of overall test analysis, both the mean PBI (0.36) and the mean p-value (0.754) for our sample are acceptable values, which means that the items on average were challenging and provided distinction between those who scored at the high end on the test and those who scored at the low end. You will need to closely examine these values for each individual item before final decisions can be made about the exam, however.

Score Distribution

A test score distribution complements the analysis of test data by providing you with a description of how the class as a whole performed on the test. A distribution helps you visualize test results and makes the scores easier to interpret. Score distributions are typically reported in a frequency table or in a graphic format.

Table 10.3 is a grouped frequency distribution that is associated with the sample data in Table 10.1. This frequency distribution groups the raw scores on the test into four-point intervals. In this distribution, you can see, for example, that six students scored between 84 and 87. This distribution provides a visual representation for interpreting the range of raw scores on a test. It enables you to visualize the significance of test analysis data such as the mean and the median and to identify how the scores on the test clustered.

TABLE 10.3   Grouped Frequency Distribution

Interval	f
92–95	1
88–91	1
84–87	6
80–83	15
76–79	24
72–75	16
68–71	13
64–67	10
60–63	2
56–59	1
52–55	3
N	92

Histogram

For many, a graphic representation of a score distribution provides the clearest visualization of a set of scores. A histogram is a bar graph of a score distribution with the height of each column indicating the number of students who scored in the interval represented by the horizontal axis. What form should the distribution of a classroom test take? The normal curve is the distribution with which most teachers are familiar. A normal curve is a symmetrical, bell-shaped distribution with the mean and median at the midpoint and scores tapering off toward each extreme as depicted in Figure 10.3. In a normal distribution, more than two-thirds of the scores will be located close to the mean; that is, plus or minus one standard deviation (while only a few scores will be at the very high or very low extremes of the distribution). Virtually all of the cases will fall within three standard deviations of the mean.

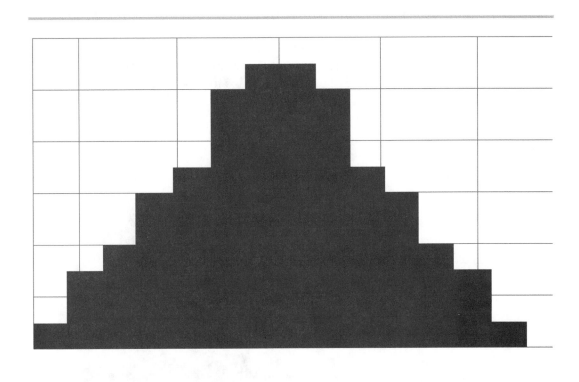

FIGURE 10.3   Normal distribution histogram

The results of most tests will approximate a normal curve when they are administered to large numbers of people (Lyman, 1998). The key word here is "large." It is most unlikely that the relatively small number of students in your class will represent a normal distribution. You should expect a normal distribution only when you test a large number of people of varying abilities. Chapter 11, "Assigning Grades," discusses why the use of the normal curve is inadvisable for classroom grading.

Refer back to Figure 10.1; it depicts a positively skewed distribution, meaning that most of the test scores are low. The shape of the distribution does not explain the cause of the problem; rather, it is a red flag that indicates that the test needs further analysis. It might mean that the test was too difficult, that the items were poorly written or confusing, that the teaching/learning activities were inadequate, that student motivation was low, or that the objectives were unrealistic. This type of distribution alerts you to investigate the cause of the problem and to take corrective action.

A negatively skewed distribution, such as the one depicted in Figure 10.2, means that most of the scores are high with only a few students at the low end. There could be several reasons for this distribution, the most desirable one being that the teaching was effective and that the students were highly motivated. It could also mean that the test was too easy or that a copy of the test or the answer key was circulating among the students. Whatever the case, further investigation is warranted.

In reality, the histograms that result from your classroom tests will not be as clear-cut as the previous samples provided here. What is important is the examination of both the frequency distribution and the histogram that represents the distribution in order to make sense of the raw scores for the test. Ask yourself what results you expected from the test and then determine what actually happened. A pretest should be positively skewed. A medication calculation test where all students are expected to pass with 90 percent correct should be negatively skewed. The score distribution for a test is a powerful tool for examining test score results.

Figure 10.4 is a histogram of the frequency distribution from Table 10.3. In the case of our sample, the score interval is four points. Note that the sample histogram illustrates that most of the scores clustered between the scores of 64 and 87 and clarifies that the mean of 75.4 represents the average score for this test.

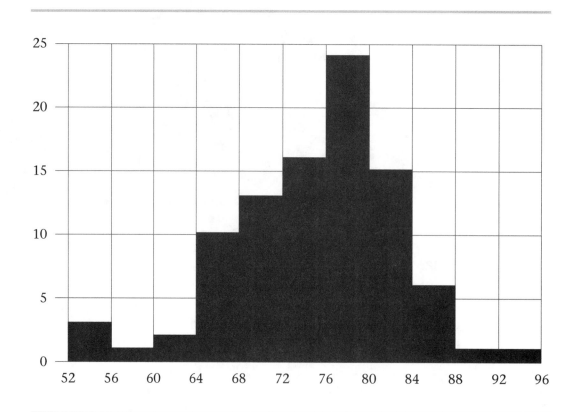

FIGURE 10.4   Histogram for sample test data

The analysis for this test is not over yet. This histogram should alert the teacher to closely examine the test. Why did 29 students attain scores of 71 or lower? What was the cause for the extremely poor performance of the six students who achieved a raw score between 52 and 63? Answers to these questions can be found in the analysis of the individual items. The analysis of the data, the frequency distribution, and the histogram (in conjunction with the analysis of the individual items) provide the best approach for determining the grade assignment for a test.

Individual Item Analysis

Once you have examined the "big picture" of the test, it is time to analyze each of the pieces. In addition to summary statistics for a test, test development software programs provide statistical analysis of each item on the test. This analysis includes the p-value and PBI for the correct answer and each of the distractors for every item. Multiple-choice classroom tests can be improved by developing a pool of good items that can be used for future tests. The statistical information from a test item analysis is an invaluable tool for both interpreting test results and improving your items for future use.

Table 10.4 provides a sample of the data that would be included in a detailed item analysis of a test. A careful review of this data will provide you with insight into the role that item data can play when you translate how items work on a test. You will see how important it is to examine all of the aspects of data analysis before making scoring decisions on a test.

Note that the p-value and the PBI for each item in the "Item Statistics" category corresponds to the p-value and PBI of the correct option in the "Option Statistics" category. For example, item #1 has a p-value of 0.71 and a PBI of 0.42—the same data as for option D (the correct answer). The response proportion figure in the "Option Statistics" category refers to the percent of students who chose each option. A comprehensive assessment requires that you examine both the difficulty (p-value) and the biserial (PBI) of each item on the test and each distractor for each item.

The difficulty level of the items determines the mean of the test. Your professional judgment is the guide for determining the acceptability of the difficulty level of the items. Ebel's suggestions for acceptability of the PBI (Table 10.2) can be used as a guide to evaluate the discrimination ability of the items. Remember, the high end of this range is a goal for which you should strive. Analysis of these data will not only help you make decisions about the test scores, but it will also guide you in improving the items for future use.

Keep in mind that you cannot look at the data in isolation. The data alerts you to look at the item; use the data as a guide. If you have a very small student sample, the data will not be as accurate as it would be with a large sample. You have a dual objective with item analysis review: one is to help you make scoring decisions about the test at hand, and the other is to improve the items in order to bank them for future use. While your judgment is the key factor, the data is a very valuable tool for guiding your judgment.

The item analysis data in Table 10.4 illustrates how this data can be used to make informed decisions about test items. Each of the first four items has an acceptable difficulty level which, if considered in isolation, would lead you to believe that the items were operating equally well on the test. Close examination of the data, however, will provide you with insight into the true functioning of the items.

Item one is an example of an item that worked well statistically. The item has a difficulty level of 0.71 and a PBI of 0.42. These findings indicate that the item discriminated very well between the high achievers and the low achievers on the test. In addition, note that each of the incorrect options has a negative PBI, which indicates

TABLE 10.4 Detailed Item Analysis

Item Statistics			Option Statistics			
Item #	p-value	PBI	Option	Response Proportion	PBI	Key
1	**0.71**	**0.42**	A	0.21	−0.30	
			B	0.03	−0.47	
			C	0.05	−0.29	
			D	**0.71**	**0.42**	**D**
2	**0.70**	**0.26**	A	0.13	−0.19	
			B	0.11	0.02	
			C	**0.70**	**0.26**	**C**
			D	0.06	−0.23	
3	**0.77**	**0.10**	A	0.07	−0.26	
			B	0.04	−0.19	
			C	0.12	0.09	
			D	**0.77**	**0.10**	**D**
4	**0.76**	**0.27**	**A**	**0.76**	**0.27**	**A**
			B	0.00	—	
			C	0.24	−0.27	
			D	0.00	—	
5	**0.258**	**−0.013**	A	0.045	−0.063	
			B	**0.258**	**−0.013**	**B**
			C	0.000	—	
			D	0.697	0.040	
6	**0.32**	**0.48**	**A**	**0.32**	**0.48**	**A**
			B	0.13	−0.24	
			C	0.18	−0.04	
			D	0.38	−0.29	
7	**1.00**	—	A	0.00	—	
			B	0.00	—	
			C	**0.00**	—	**C**
			D	0.00	—	

that the low-scoring students chose the distractors more frequently than the high-scoring students. This picture is exactly what you want to have for your items: the correct answer in an acceptable difficulty range with a high positive biserial and all of the distractors having a negative biserial.

Item two has approximately the same p-value as item one. While the biserial of the item is acceptable, however, this item was not as statistically effective as item one because option B (a distractor) has a positive biserial. A positive biserial means that high-achieving students chose the option. Perhaps the distractor was confusing or tricky. In any event, this information is a red flag for you to take a closer look to determine whether there is a problem with the item. When you examine the actual item, you might decide that the test scores should be adjusted to accept option B as a correct answer. If you look only at the difficulty level for this item, you would miss the problem with distractor B.

Another example of the problems that result from restricting your data review to the difficulty level of the items is exemplified by item three. While the item's difficulty level could be considered in the acceptable range, distractor C has a positive biserial and the correct answer (D) has very poor discrimination ability. This item should be carefully reviewed and option C considered for acceptance as a correct answer on this test before being edited and banked.

One goal of effective item writing is to develop plausible distractors that will be attractive to the uninformed students. In order for a distractor to contribute to an item, someone must choose it. When no one chooses an option, it is considered a non-distractor. Item four has two non-distractors. No one chose either option B or D. Although the item has an acceptable difficulty level and it discriminated in the marginal range, it was effectively a true-false item. Both options that were not chosen should be revised before the item is banked.

Item five is an example of an item where the correct answer has a negative biserial. In addition, option C was not chosen, and item D has a positive biserial and was chosen by the majority of the students. These findings indicate that the students were confused and were probably guessing. Perhaps the item is miskeyed. Even if it is miskeyed, however, it has very weak discrimination power and needs to be revised. Based on the data of this item, you should review it and consider discarding it from this test and revising it extensively before entering it into your item bank.

Look carefully at item six. If you were only to look at the difficulty level for this item, you might discard it because it is so difficult. The data indicates, however, that the item has excellent discrimination capability and that all three distractors have negative biserials. Perhaps the item is a challenging one that enables the test to identify high-achieving students. In order to determine the true value of this item, you will need to keep the data in mind while you review the item itself.

Item seven illustrates how an item that is too easy cannot discriminate. Everyone answered this question correctly. No one chose any of the options. This item might be too easy, or maybe it is testing a concept that you want to be certain that the students understand. Items such as this one must be carefully reviewed before they are entered into an item bank. Chapter 12, "Instituting Item Banking and Test Development Software," carries this discussion further by presenting actual examples of items and demonstrating how to combine quantitative and qualitative analysis to improve your items.

It is clear from this sample item analysis review that the statistical data provided in most software reports can provide a valuable tool for making scoring decisions and for improving your items for future use. An understanding of the basic concepts will go a long way toward helping you translate this data. Follow the steps outlined in Figure 10.5 to guide you through the test and item analysis process.

Overall Analysis

- Check data for completeness
- Assess the relationship of the mean and the median
- Examine the relationship of the mean to the passing standard
- Check the score range and SD
- Examine the reliability coefficient
- Determine the SEM
- Examine the mean p-value
- Evaluate the mean biserial
- Examine the score frequency distribution
- Assess the test's histogram

Individual Item Analysis

- Assess each item's p-value
- Examine each item's PBI
- Identify that the key has a positive PBI
- Identify if any distractor has a positive PBI
- Identify distractors that were not chosen
- Review items that violate minimum standards and consider discarding from test
- Revise items based on data before entering them into an item bank

---

FIGURE 10.5   Statistical test analysis

Assigning Test Scores

Once you have collected data from qualitative, statistical, and student review, you can assign scores to an exam. While you might decide to discard an item or accept more than one correct answer for a question, it is usually best not to add points to individual exams. This practice, referred to as scaling scores, is discussed further in Chapter 11, "Assigning Grades."

Flawed Items

Items that are seriously flawed should not be counted as part of the final test score. Eliminating poorly functioning items from a test can increase the test's reliability coefficient. Kehoe (1995) provides an example of how eliminating seven items that had PBIs below 0.20 from a test of 30 items with a reliability coefficient of 0.79 resulted in a 23-item test with a reliability coefficient of 0.88.

It is impossible to determine whether an item is seriously flawed based on either quantitative or qualitative analysis alone. In order to fairly assess the items, you must include the overall test data, the item analysis data, the student review, and your qualitative review of the items in question. If you conclude that an item is flawed based on your comprehensive analysis, you might decide to accept more than one option as the correct answer for the item or to eliminate the item from the test. It is important to note that because of measurement error, giving the benefit of the doubt to the students is usually the fairest approach.

Flawed items should be revised before they are entered into the item bank in order to ensure that they are not reused in the defective condition. Flawed items often have the potential to become very effective items. Careful editing that considers the qualitative and quantitative analysis and that incorporates student comments can assist you with transforming these items into items that contribute to valid and reliable measurement instruments.

Returning Scores to Students

Teachers must carefully consider the issue of confidentiality when returning scores to students. Several test development programs provide individual score reports that can be confidentially distributed to students. Many schools have the ability to confidentially distribute scores on the Web. If your school's practice is to post student grades, be careful to assign secret identification numbers to each student.

Another important consideration is timeliness. All too often, teachers assign strict deadlines for assignment submissions, yet they are very lax with returning the same assignments in a timely manner. While careful consideration of grade assignment requires time, students should not be required to wait until the feedback from an exam or written assignment is meaningless. In the interest of fairness, teachers should set a return deadline with the student and adhere to that deadline.

Summary

Systematic test and item analysis procedures ensure the fairness and accuracy of individual items and the test as a whole. It is impossible to evaluate the effectiveness of an item on a test without examining all of the relevant data. Statistical test and item analysis data provide the essential tools for objective review of test results. This chapter provides actual examples of test analysis data to illustrate how this data can be used for objective interpretation of test results. While your first attempt at conducting these analyses will be time consuming, the procedure will become streamlined as you become more proficient and as you are able to incorporate "proven" items from your item bank in your exams.

11 Assigning Grades

> "What a mark means is determined not only by how it was
> defined when the marking system was adopted, but also, and
> perhaps more importantly, by the way it is actually used."
>
> —Robert Ebel

Grades matter. Classroom grades represent a high-stakes situation for many reasons. They are the basis for decisions about progression in a program. They determine who graduates. They send an authoritative message about the quality of a student's work to employers and graduate schools. Because of the powerful influence that classroom grades have on the lives of students, it is imperative that the assignment of grades is based on high-quality information (Nitko, 1996).

A grade is a label that represents a summary of a student's achievement of the course content and instructional objectives. There is no simple grading system. Grading is a complex process that is subject to error because course grades are derived from a combination of scores from instruments that are all subject to measurement error. Because grades have such serious implications, every assignment that has a direct impact on a student's course grade must be a valid and reliable instrument and be measured with extreme objectivity. Only by having a clear understanding of the factors that influence grading can you reduce error and develop a fair and objective system for assigning grades.

Grading Principles

Grades represent the culmination of the assessment process. They symbolize the quality of a student's performance. You will note that the principles of grading incorporate the elements of the assessment process that have been presented in this book. These

181

elements are links in the processes; they contribute individually, and as a whole, to quality assessment practices. The process of grading is only as strong as the weakest link in this process.

No grading system is perfect. It is important to acknowledge that grades are influenced by subjectivity and measurement error. Only by following a systematic assessment plan can you have confidence that your instructional process is valid and that the grades you assign represent a fair evaluation of student performance.

Experts agree that a grading plan must be based on the principles of grading (Airasian, 1997; Haladyna, 1999; Linn & Gronlund, 2000; Nitko, 1996; Ory & Ryan, 1993). These principles include the following:

- **Grades are important.** Grades send powerful messages that have significant impact on the lives of students.

- **Grading should be based on course objectives and content.** Grades should be based on the same objectives that guide instruction. If you follow the assessment guidelines presented in this book, your classroom tests will be based on the content and instructional objectives of your course.

- **Grading should be objective.** While subjective grading is dependent on a teacher's judgment, objective grading leads to the same result no matter who assigns the grade. Every measurement instrument that contributes to a grade must meet this standard for objectivity. To meet this criterion, teachers have to be willing to admit when they have made a mistake. They must be able to recognize, for example, when an item on a test might have misled students or might have had two feasible answers.

- **Grading should be based on credible assessment.** Validity and reliability provide the foundation for credible assessment and fair grading. The more confidence you have in the measurements you use, the more confidence you will have in the grades that you assign. At the same time, objective grades require adequate evidence. You cannot make valid decisions based on insufficient evidence.

- **Grading must be confidential.** Teachers are prevented by law from discussing or divulging the grades of students who are 18 years old or older without the written permission of the student. Care must be taken to protect student privacy during all phases of the grading process. Even the posting of grades can pose a threat to confidentiality if a system is used that enables students to decode each other's grades.

- **Grading policies should be clearly written and presented on the first day of class.** Most institutions require faculty to have clearly written grading criteria in the course syllabus. You should also discuss the plan with the students and clarify any misconceptions. These practices are essential to enable students to plan strategies for success.

- **Grades influence students' incentive to learn.** Grades are intended to reflect what a student has learned. Haladyna (1999) asserts that although grades are extrinsic motivators, a well-defined grading method will increase student motivation and will propel the students toward more learning, eventually leading to intrinsic motivation.

While high grades motivate students, lower-than-expected grades or grades that are perceived as unfair can seriously diminish student motivation. Instead of prompting greater effort, low grades, especially those that are perceived as unfair, might cause students to withdraw from learning. Most importantly, there are no studies to support using low grades as punishment (Guskey, 1994).

While you want to provide incentives for students, fairness does not require that you assign high grades to all students. In fact, lowering standards to ensure high grades decreases student motivation and effort and reduces the validity of your grade assignments. Fairness in grading requires that you set standards that can be realistically achieved by students if they work hard (Airasian, 1997).

Philosophy of Grading

The process of grading requires teachers to develop a plan that is in harmony with their personal grading philosophy. Grading decisions are based not only on established principles, but also on a teacher's beliefs about the teaching-learning process (Frisbie & Waltman, 1992). These principles and beliefs are incorporated into a grading philosophy, which guides a teacher's grading plan.

Before you can develop a plan, you need to identify your grading philosophy. Frisbie & Waltman (1992, p. 36) present a series of nine "should" questions for teachers to answer when examining their beliefs about grading. These questions have no right or wrong answers; reasonable people will disagree. These are questions that must be answered to help you to articulate your grading philosophy, however. Your answers must be consistent with one another if you are to form a solid basis for your grading plan.

1. What meaning should each grade symbol carry?

The meaning of each grade must be clearly understood by both students and the teacher. This question has two components: What areas of student achievement are included in the grade? How do the symbols reflect the degree of student achievement?

Although some institutions use numerical grades, letters are used most frequently to represent the degree of student performance on a scale that ranges from excellent to failing. Pluses and/or minuses are often used with the letters to further delineate the level of student performance. The parent institution usually determines the letters that can be used for grade assignment and the definition of each letter assignment. Table 11.1 presents a sample of an institution's grading scale.

The parent institution usually mandates how these letter grades are translated into numerical values so that a *grade-point average* (GPA) can be calculated for each student. The numerical values associated with each letter are frequently referred to as quality points, as the sample in Table 11.2 illustrates. It is important that the grading symbols and quality point equivalents are consistent across departments in a college or university so that student GPAs will be consistent.

TABLE 11.1   Sample grading scale

A   Outstanding

A-   Superior

B+   Very Good

B   Good

B-   Above Average

C+   Upper Level of Average

C   Average

C-   Poor

D   Minimal Pass

F   Fail

P   Pass

W   Withdraw

TABLE 11.2   Sample quality point index

Grade	Quality Points
A	4.0
A-	3.7
B+	3.5
B	3.0
B-	2.7
C+	2.5
C	2.0
C-	1.7
D	1.0
F	0

The GPA is computed by multiplying the credit value for each course by the number of points associated with the grade earned to obtain the total quality points for each course. The total quality points for each course are then added together, and this sum is divided by the total number of credit hours in order to obtain the scholastic average, or GPA, for each student. Table 11.3 provides an example of how grades are translated into quality points to calculate a student's GPA. The GPA is used to set a standard for retention and graduation. It is also used to rank students and is an important factor for employment and graduate school admission.

TABLE 11.3 Sample GPA Calculation

Course	Grade	Quality Points	Credit Hours	Total Quality Points
Hist 101	A	4.0	3	12.0
Soc 101	C+	2.5	3	7.5
Eng 101	B	3.0	3	9.0
Art 101	B+	3.5	3	10.5
Total			**12**	**39**
GPA				**3.25**

The GPA is determined by dividing the total quality points by the total credit hours ($39 \div 12 = 3.25$).

Every college or university publishes a course catalog in which the description of the letter grades and their associated quality points are clearly described, along with the school's academic policies. The school's catalog constitutes a contract with the students; it spells out the academic requirements for receiving a degree from the institution.

While your parent institution might determine what grading symbol you must use, individual departments or faculty members are usually responsible for determining the achievement components to be considered and the level of performance that is required for translation of student achievement into a specific grade symbol. Will your grade assignment include only achievement of the defined content and instructional objectives, or will you consider class participation and effort as part of the grade? What level of understanding does a grade of B represent? What does "good" mean? Before you can assign a grade, you must determine what the grading symbols mean. Your grading plan will incorporate your answers to these nine questions.

2. What should failure mean?

It is a difficult task to assign a failing grade to a student. The negative consequences of the F grade create an emotional atmosphere that most teachers would prefer to avoid (Frisbie & Waltman, 1992). Other grades can also have negative significance. For example, a grade of D might be unsatisfactory for progression in a program or might not count toward graduation. Nitko (1996) points out that your answer to this question should be consistent with your perception of the meaning of all grades. Nitko suggests establishing minimum standards of performance on the curriculum and learning outcomes and assigning a failing grade to those students who consistently perform below those minimum standards.

3. What elements of performance should be incorporated in a grade?

Grades should be assigned objectively. Once you decide what a grade symbolizes, all extraneous information should be kept out of the grading decision. In other words, if grades are designed to reflect achievement levels of the course content and objectives, only achievement activities should be included in the grade decision.

Components such as effort and class participation should be excluded from grading criteria. These factors are far too arbitrary and subjective to be included in an objective grade. It is unfair to grade a student on what could very well be a personality issue. How can you objectively assign a grade to effort? Is an unassertive student necessarily uninvolved in the class presentation? Unless constructs such as effort and assertiveness are operationally defined and included in your course objectives, it is unfair to include these factors in your grade assignments. It is particularly unfair to use a subjective evaluation of a student's class participation to decrease a student's overall grade.

If you want students to participate in class, an assignment such as an oral presentation that is graded with objective criteria that are shared with the students is one fair way to assign a grade. An objective grade is one that a student can figure out based on the course syllabus, without additional subjective input from the teacher (Haladyna, 1999).

4. How should the grades in a class be distributed?

Is there a limit to the number of A grades you will assign? Will C be the average grade? What percentage of failing grades is acceptable? Although it is unusual, some institutions do have policies about grade distribution that will influence the grades that you assign. Even when there is no written policy, professors who assign a large number of high or low grades might be questioned by school administration about their grading policy. If your grade distribution is consistent with your answers to the first three questions, you will be able to justify your grade assignments.

5. What components should go into a final grade?

Your grading plan will specify the components that will determine the final grade for a course. As Frisbe & Waltman (1992) point out, the separate scores that are combined to determine the final course grade must reflect the meaning that you have assigned for the grade symbols. Moreover, each assessment task that contributes to a grade must reflect the elements of performance that you designated in question three. If your definition of the grade components includes only achievement in the areas of course content and instructional objectives, then components such as class participation and effort should be excluded from the final grade.

6. How should the components of the grade be combined?

Once the components of a grade are determined, you must decide how to weight the scores derived from each of these measurements to determine a composite grade. Will each component be worth an equal percentage of the grade, or should some be counted more heavily? The answer to this question will determine how you calculate the composite grade.

7. What method should be used to assign grades?

After you combine the measurement scores, you must assign final grades to the students. Frisbe & Waltman (1992) remind us that your method of grade assignment must reflect your definition of the meaning of the grade symbols. If your answer to question one indicates that grades reflect degrees of student achievement of the content and instructional objectives of the course, it would be illogical to assign grades based on a curve. Methods for assigning grades are discussed later in this chapter.

8. Should borderline cases be reviewed?

How will you handle the situation where a composite grade puts a student right on the borderline between passing and failing? How close to passing must a student's composite score be before it is rounded up? Will you allow students to submit work for extra credit to raise a borderline grade? If all of the grades are particularly low, will you add points or "scale" the scores?

Previous discussion has established that all measurements contain error. Therefore, will you look only at a student's observed score, or will you take the standard error of measurement into account when considering what the student's true score might be? Many experts, including Nitko (1996), recommend giving the student the benefit of the doubt by collecting additional information to help you decide whether the student's true score is greater than the observed score. In fact, Nitko recommends that educators give the higher grade when there is serious doubt about whether a student is above or below the boundary for passing.

9. What other factors can influence the philosophy of grading?

The parent institution for your nursing program has considerable authority in determining the academic policies that you must follow when assigning grades. Issues such as grade distribution, course credit, and degree requirements will have an impact on your grading philosophy. You have to be cognizant of these issues when you develop your plan.

Some nursing programs use a uniform system of grading. This approach makes sense as long as it allows for differences in instructional approaches. Teachers should always have flexibility when deciding on the components of a grade. When a uniform system is devised, the faculty must come to a consensus on all of the issues surrounding the development of a grading philosophy. Each of these nine questions must be addressed as a group. Agreeing on a grading policy is not an easy task for a faculty group, but it is essential for assuring fairness—particularly for courses that consist of several sections.

Another issue that faculty must face when assigning grades is to consider the criteria applied in other departments. It is unfair to punish nursing students with a stringent grading policy or reward them with a very lenient grading policy that diminishes their standing in the greater college community. While it is very important to maintain your academic standards, you should consider the implications of your grade assignments on the GPAs of nursing students as compared to other students in your college or university.

Developing a Grading Plan

Calculating course grades is not just a mathematical exercise; it is an expression of your philosophy. A sound grading plan incorporates your philosophy with the principles of grading to assign grades. The model you use for weighting the components of the final grade communicates to your students what you think is important; it tells them where they should put their efforts (Walvoord & Anderson, 1998). Regardless of which model you use to establish your grading system, the standard should be established before the plan is initiated. In fact, the plan should be communicated to the students at the outset of the course so that they will know how to focus their efforts.

Weighting Components of a Grade

The initial step in the grading process is to determine what components will be included in the grade and how the components will be combined to produce a composite grade. Every assessment of achievement is not necessarily of equal importance in the determination of a grade; you need to develop a system to assign weights to the various components. The amount of weight that you allot for each component will be based on your judgment of the significance of the component in the grading scheme. Nitko (1996) suggests that you make a list of all the assessment tasks for the semester, decide how each task relates to the course content and objectives, and then assign a weight based on how important each task is in relation to the composite grade.

A grade represents a judgment about a student's achievement. In order to judge that achievement, a standard must be identified against which to compare student performance. Once you have decided how your grading components will be weighted, you must determine which framework you will use to serve as the basis for assigning student grades. The two most commonly used are the absolute standard and the relative standard.

Absolute Standard

An absolute standard or a criterion-referenced standard compares a student's performance to a prespecified standard of performance (Gronlund, 1993) and assigns grades by comparing student performance with the objectives to be attained and the content to be mastered. With this model, grades are based solely on the standards. Students who demonstrate a high level of achievement receive high grades without regard to how well other students perform (Nitko, 1996). When this standard is applied, all of the students could theoretically receive a grade of A. Of course, it is also theoretically possible that every student could receive a grade of F. Remember that all of the aspects of the assessment process work in concert, however. Careful design of your measurement instruments will ensure that the items discriminate and that you have a range of scores that reflect levels of student achievement. It will also ensure that you have a valid and reliable basis for determining grade assignments based on your predetermined set of criteria.

Absolute grading methods require that the performance standards be clearly described and that the measurement instruments that comprise the composite score yield valid and reliable information about student achievement in relation to the standards. The content and instructional objectives that are established at the outset of the course comprise the standards that are used to determine student grades. If you follow the guidelines described in this book to establish a systematic assessment plan, your classroom exams will provide trustworthy information about student performance related to those standards.

The model you use to translate the scores into a letter grade is a matter of personal choice, although the choice should be consistent for all sections of the same course. Whichever model you choose, the criteria must be explained to students and should be included in the course syllabus.

FIXED PERCENT SCALE   The formula for the fixed percent method includes the weighting that you have assigned to each assessment task. An illustration of how you will weight the grades, such as that in Table 11.4, should be included in the course syllabus.

TABLE 11.4   Sample Grade Weighting

Pharmacology Quiz	10%
Unit I Exam	20%
Unit II Exam	20%
Nursing Process Paper	20%
Final Exam	30%

With this method, a percent correct score is determined for every component of the assessment composite, including exams, term papers, and presentations. Each component is given a percent correct, which represents the percent of the maximum score that the student received on the component (Nitko, 1996). For example, a student who earns a score of 46 out of 50 possible points on an exam would receive a score of 92 percent. Table 11.5 illustrates how the percent score for each component is multiplied by the weight assigned to it, and the products for all components are summed to determine the final score.

By using a grade book that has a column for calculating the weight of each grade as the semester progresses, the calculation of the composite grade will be less tedious at the end of the course. If you keep your grades by hand, it is a good idea to keep the weighted grade figure in red or in some color that contrasts with the percent score. Table 11.5 indicates the weighted grade in a bold font.

TABLE 11.5 Sample Calculation of Grades Using the Fixed Percent Method

SCORES

	Pharmacology Quiz		Unit I Exam		Unit II Exam		Nursing Process Paper		Final Exam		Grade
Weights	10% (.1)		20% (.2)		20% (.2)		20% (.2)		30% (.3)		
	CS	WS	CS	WS	CS	WS	CS	WS	CS	WS	
T. Bass	85	**8.5**	80	**16**	90	**18**	75	**15**	85	**25.5**	**83%**
A. Crew	90	**9.0**	88	**17.6**	84	**16.8**	90	**18**	86	**25.8**	**87.2%**
G. Lamb	95	**9.5**	90	**18**	82	**16.4**	80	**16**	90	**27**	**86.9%**

Multiply each component percent score (CS) by its percentage weighting to obtain the weighted score (WS) for each component. Add the weighted scores for each component to obtain the composite grade.

You can enter your grades into an electronic spreadsheet and have the program do the calculations for you. A simple spreadsheet is easy to develop, and most schools have resources to help you gain expertise in using the computer software programs that produce spreadsheets. There are also several electronic grade book programs available that facilitate the process of calculating grades. The better ones offer you several options for specifying rules for assigning grades and also provide the ability to maintain class rosters, keep track of attendance, and prepare summary grade reports for groups and individual students. Several of the test development software programs that are discussed in Chapter 12, "Instituting Item Banking and Test Development Software," link to grade books that interface with the testing program to automatically import scores and calculate grades based on your grading plan.

It is important to recognize that the relationship between the percent composite score and the scale for determining a grade is a subjective process. Assigning grades requires synthesizing a great deal of information into a single symbol, and the cutoff between grade categories is always arbitrary (Guskey, 1994). The more systematic your grading plan, the more objective your grade assignments.

While the parent institution defines the symbols—usually a letter—to be used for grading and the quality points assigned to each letter, the translation of the percent composite score to a letter is usually left to the individual department or faculty members. In these situations, the faculty determines the achievement levels that correspond to the letters identified by the parent institution. While faculty should always have the authority to determine the components of a composite score, there are situations where faculty must follow the guidelines of the college or university for translating a composite percent correct score to a letter grade, as is shown in Table 11.6. Whatever

the case, it is important that students are fully aware of the grading scale and its interpretations.

TABLE 11.6   Sample Translation of a Composite Percent Correct Score to a Letter Grade

Grade Assignment

Composite Percent Score	Grade
90–100%	A
80–89%	B
70–79%	C
60–69%	D
<60%	F

TOTAL POINTS SCALE   With the total points approach, the composite grade for
the student is the total of the points that the student receives. Each assessment task is
assigned a number of points based on the weight assigned to it, and the point total at
the end of the course is translated into a composite grade based on the number of
points required for the grade. Keeping the maximum number of points at 100 or 1,000
makes this system easier for the student to understand. Table 11.7 illustrates how the
sample grade weighting from Table 11.4 would translate to a total points scale.

TABLE 11.7   Sample Total Points Scale

Pharmacology Quiz	100
Unit I Exam	200
Unit II Exam	200
Nursing Process Paper	200
Final Exam	<u>300</u>
Maximum Points	1000

Table 11.8 illustrates how grades can be calculated by using a total points scale.

The relationship between the composite score derived from a total points scale score
and the scale for determining a letter grade is just as arbitrary as the fixed percent scale,
as is shown in Table 11.9. The grade symbols determined by the parent institution
define the grade range and the quality points assigned to each grade. The question you
must answer is, "How many total points correspond to each letter grade?"

TABLE 11.8   Sample Calculation of Grades Using the Total Points Method

SCORES

	Pharmacology Quiz		Unit I Exam		Unit II Exam		Nursing Process Paper		Final Exam		Total Points
Points	100		200		200		200		300		
	CS	WS	CS	WS	CS	WS	CS	WS	CS	WS	
T. Bass	85	**85**	80	**160**	90	**180**	75	**150**	85	**255**	**830**
A. Crew	90	**90**	88	**176**	84	**168**	90	**180**	86	**258**	**872**
G. Lamb	95	**95**	90	**180**	82	**164**	80	**160**	90	**270**	**869**

Multiply each component percent score (CS) by its number of points to obtain the weighted score (WS) for each component. Add the weighted scores for each component to obtain the total number of points.

TABLE 11.9   Sample Translation of Total Points Composite to a Letter Grade

Grade Assignment

Total Points Composite Score	Grade
900–1000	A
800–899	B
700–799	C
600–699	D
<600	F

Relative Standard

Assigning grades on a relative basis, also referred to as norm-referenced grading, assigns student grades based on their ranking compared to other students in the class based on a combination of assessment results. With this approach to grading, students are ranked in order of performance, or graded on a "curve"—whereby the teacher predetermines the percentage of students who will receive each grade. The "curve" is the curve of the normal distribution.

Grading on the normal curve yields a percentage of A's and F's and B's and D's so that the number of high grades is balanced by an equal number of low grades. Worthen, Borg, and White describe that the most common method used to determine letter grades based on the normal curve is based on the mean and standard deviation of the test. They explain that if the test results yield a normal curve, then grades would be distributed as follows (1993, p. 385):

A = approximately 7 percent (1.5 standard deviations above the mean)

B = approximately 24 percent (0.5 to 1.5 standard deviations above the mean)

C = approximately 38 percent (0.5 standard deviations above the mean to 0.5 standard deviations below the mean)

D = approximately 24 percent (0.5 to 1.5 standard deviations below the mean)

F = approximately 7 percent (1.5 standard deviations below the mean)

This method presents several problems for assigning classroom grades. First, classroom measurements are unlikely to yield a normal distribution of scores. When teachers who want to use a relative standard for grading recognize that classroom groups are too small for assessment results to resemble a normal curve, they often use their judgment to establish a grading curve that ensures that there is a distribution of grades. These judgments arbitrarily establish quotas for each grade to be given, as shown in Table 11.10.

TABLE 11.10   Example of Arbitrary Assignment of Grade Quotas

Grade	Percent of Students
A	10
B	25
C	50
D	10
F	5

Another problem with relative grade assignment is that the normative group is the students in a given class. In other words, the standard is totally dependent upon the composition of the class with no indication of actual student achievement. Therefore, a student's grade depends more on the other students in the class than on how well the student has mastered the material (Worthen, Borg, & White, 1993). Because the standard is based on best and worst performances, some students will receive good grades regardless of their level of knowledge, and some will receive low grades no matter what their level of achievement (Popham, 1999).

In the example illustrated in Table 11.10, the teacher has predetermined that only 10 percent of the class will receive a grade of A while 5 percent would be destined for failure. With this plan, in a class of 30 students, only three would receive an A regardless of the mastery level of the individual students. If the best student in this group had a composite score of only 40 out of a possible 100 points, the student would receive a grade of A. On the other hand, if the lowest student in a group of high-achieving students received 85 out of a possible 100 points, that student would necessarily receive a grade of F. Walvoord and Anderson (1998) associate grading on the curve with focusing the teacher's role on awarding grades by formula rather than on rewarding student learning with earned and deserved grades.

Most experts agree that educationally sound grading should be based on a student's level of achievement, not on some relative ranking in a group. Haladyna (1999) maintains that the relative standard should never be used for classroom grading because it is associated with so many negative consequences. These consequences include the following:

- Establishing unhealthy competition among the top students for the limited number of A grades

- Reducing cooperation among students at all levels who recognize that their success is dependent upon the performance of their classmates

- Ensuring that some students will fail no matter what their level of mastery

- Demoralizing those students who are ranked at the bottom of the group and undermining their learning efforts

Refer to Table 11.11 for a comparison of absolute and reference standard grading

TABLE 11.11   Comparison of Absolute and Referenced Grading

Absolute Standard	Referenced Standard
Predetermines criteria for grade assignment	Predetermines quotas for each grade assignment
Bases grade on student achievement	Bases grade on comparison of students
Dependent on achievement of standard	Dependent on composition of class.
Can be designed to foster student cooperation	Establishes unhealthy student competition
Enables all students to pass	Ensures that some students will fail

Pass/Fail Grading

Most colleges and universities enable students to take courses on a pass/fail basis. Usually, the number of times a student can opt for the pass/fail grade is limited, and the pass/fail grade is not included in the calculation of the student's GPA. Some experts maintain that pass/fail grading encourages students to experiment, to take courses that they otherwise would avoid for fear of decreasing their GPA. Others argue that the pass/fail option discourages high achievement and encourages students to direct their study efforts at merely passing. Usually, this option is not offered for courses in the student's major. The policy for pass/fail grading, which varies widely among schools, is always stated in the official course catalog.

Many nursing programs use the pass/fail option for grading clinical practice. When nursing students are expected to demonstrate achievement of all of the objectives measured in a practice setting, pass or fail is an appropriate grade assignment. Additionally, clinical evaluation is prone to subjectivity. Even with the most objective assessment instrument, it can be very difficult to distinguish between different levels of proficiency among students in the clinical practice setting.

It is beyond the scope of this discussion to review criteria for clinical evaluation. The clinical evaluation instrument, however, must be congruent with the objectives and content of the overall course. In fact, several of your learning outcomes might be conducive only to clinical evaluation (as Tables 3.3 and 4.4 illustrate).

The critical concern with the pass/fail grading option is that the course follows all of the assessment guidelines. When a student elects the pass/fail option, the professor does not necessarily know of this election, so the student is graded on the same basis as other students in the class who elect to receive a grade. It is the registrar who converts the grade to pass or fail. When a course is given on a pass/fail basis to an entire class, the instructor must be careful to ensure that the grading criteria are as precise as the criteria for a graded course. A grade plan should be developed, and the student's composite grade should reflect a score above the passing level based on the standard in order to receive a passing score.

Adjusting Grades

In an attempt to increase the fairness of classroom grade assignments and to give students the maximum opportunity to demonstrate achievement, teachers have devised a variety of methods to enhance classroom grades. You might want to increase the grade assignments if, for example, the semester exams were more difficult than you intended. While you do not want to make grade changes frivolously, it is better to make changes than to assign grades that are unfair (Airasian, 1997).

Scaling Grades

While curving is based on norm referencing, which is not recommended for classroom grading, scaling is derived from criterion-referenced testing (Trice, 2000). When grades are scaled, a certain number of set points are added to each student's score. While the number of failures might be the impetus for increasing grades, the shape of the grade curve is not. Reviewing test and item analysis and examining the appropriateness of the expected performance standard will help you to determine whether, and how many, points should be added to the scores.

Most teachers are very concerned with grade inflation. Assigning grades requires a "balancing act." A careful analysis of each assessment component of your grades will help you determine whether the final grades need to be adjusted. The best approach is to wait until the end of the course to make grade changes. If, for example, you added points to exam one, that exam would have a greater weight in the final course grade. In order to maintain the designated weighting of the components, determine the grades based on the predetermined weighting and adjust the final composite grade.

Keep in mind that adjusting grades is a subjective process, and fairness does not mean that everyone gets a high grade. Remember, lowering standards to assign higher grades will discourage student effort and decrease the validity of the grades (Airasian, 1997). Your discretion is essential. Before you alter the grades, carefully examine the qualitative and quantitative analyses of all of the exams to determine how well they measure the course objectives and learning outcomes, and apply the adjustment equally for all students.

Giving Extra Credit

The practice of giving extra credit is widespread at all levels of education. Extra credit can assume forms such as allowing students to redo a paper or write a report for a unit on which they performed poorly. Extra credit items can also be included on an exam as either constructed- or selected-response items to allow all students the opportunity to increase their grades. As long as the extra-credit assignment addresses the content and objectives of the course, it is an acceptable method for assessing student achievement. As Trice (2000) humorously points out, giving extra credit for after-class janitorial activities would be a questionable practice.

Remember, assessment procedures should be designed to give students every opportunity to demonstrate attainment of the course objectives. Just be certain that extra-credit activities do not unfairly alter the weighting of the course components and that they are equally available to all students.

Dropping the Lowest Grade

Discounting the students' lowest test grade when determining the final composite score has advantages and disadvantages. While the practice enables students to have "a bad day," Trice (2000) points out that it disconnects assessment from the course objectives because when teachers drop a grade, they are saying that the students do not need to meet some of the course objectives. It also alters the weighting of the course content and objectives. Trice proposes that a better practice is to allow students to take a makeup exam on the content on which they performed poorly. A good application for extra credit would be to allow students to complete one extra-credit assignment in the area of their weakest test score.

Usually, extra-credit opportunities and the option for dropping the lowest grade are clearly spelled out in the course syllabus. The instructional process is not one that you should set in stone, however. If a grading standard or criterion turns out to be inappropriate or unfair, it should be changed (Airasian, 1997). While you cannot make your grading criteria more stringent at the end of a course than what you have designated in the syllabus, students will never object to having an added opportunity to demonstrate their attainment of objectives. Grades are important to students. Failing students are not the only ones who are concerned with extra-credit assignments. High-achieving students have "bad days," too. The key concern is to apply all criteria fairly and equally to all students.

Summary

An equitable grading plan is based on grading principles and the teacher's philosophy of grading. Classroom grades have serious implications for students; therefore, teachers must be aware of these implications and the variables that affect grading in order to determine what grading system will best suit the needs of their students. Although the selection of a grading framework is up to the teacher, experts generally agree that a norm-referenced system is inappropriate for classroom grading. It is important that teachers maintain flexibility, give thoughtful consideration to each of the decisions that must be made when developing a scheme for classroom grading, and share the final plan with the students at the outset of the course.

A grade is only as fair as the instructional process on which it is based. The ultimate goal of a systematic assessment plan is the assignment of grades that fairly reflect student mastery of the content and objectives of a course. Each component of the assessment plan plays an important role in achieving this outcome. The guidelines presented in this book build on each other and work together in the assessment process to create an overall plan that ultimately results in fair grade assignment. Appendix E, "Steps for Implementing a Systematic Assessment Plan," delineates the steps for implementing a systematic assessment plan.

12 Instituting Item Banking and Test Development Software

"Change is not made without inconvenience, even from worse to better."

—Richard Hooker

Computer technology is changing the face of educational assessment at every level. Only a few years ago very few could afford to take advantage of computerized testing. Fortunately, the current widespread availability of personal computers, coupled with the proliferation of sophisticated test development software that is designed to be user-friendly, has made electronic item banking a workable reality. The potential for streamlining the process of preparing valid and reliable multiple-choice classroom exams is now readily available to classroom teachers. The software, which is reasonably priced, offers educators the best possible approach for ensuring the quality and objective fairness of their classroom assessments.

The time has arrived for every educator who uses multiple-choice classroom exams to institute item banking/test development software. If you are having difficulty convincing your administration to fund the purchase of the hardware and software required to initiate computer-assisted test development, this chapter will help you to argue the case. Even if you are fully funded and have administration's support, you may meet with some faculty resistance when you introduce a software testing program. Resistance accompanies all change. Those who are not comfortable with computer technology will be the most resistant. The important thing to remember is that these programs are only tools; in fact, most programs are designed to require a minimum of computer ability. Think of the technology as simply replacing your pen, index card, calculator, and file cabinet. The software does not create the test; it facilitates your work and allows you to create the best possible assessment instrument. While there is a learning curve associated with acquiring computer skills, the payoff is well worth the effort.

The key to a smooth transition from manual test development to a computerized testing program is careful planning. The goal of this chapter is threefold: to demonstrate that developing an item bank and implementing test development software is the most efficient means for actualizing a systematic assessment plan; to improve your skills at editing and updating items based on analysis data; and to help you to identify your priorities when selecting test development software. This information will provide the basis for developing a plan to streamline the process of implementing a computerized testing program. Today's software programs offer such advantages for test development that educators can no longer afford to ignore the potential of technology.

Establishing an Item Bank

As defined in Chapter 2, "The Language of Assessment," an item bank is an organized collection of accessible test items designed to facilitate the preparation of future exams. Item banking is an essential tool for the development of valid and reliable multiple-choice classroom exams. An item bank allows you to "deposit" items that can be withdrawn as needed (Rudner, 1998), thereby eliminating the need to write all new items for every exam. It is also a valuable tool for developing make-up exams and a helpful asset for junior faculty. A well-developed item bank supplies new faculty with a valuable resource for developing tests and also provides a working example of quality item writing.

As the previous chapters have illustrated, test development is a time-consuming process that requires considerable effort, a time commitment that you certainly would rather not expend every semester. While most teachers recycle their multiple-choice test items, a well-planned item bank provides a systematic approach for using item analysis data to improve your items while you save them and, as a result, improve your classroom assessments. The effort that you invest in developing items can be "banked" in an organized manner for future use.

Until a few years ago, experts who advocated item banking for classroom multiple-choice test development usually advised writing each item on an individual index card with codes for categories such as course content and objective. Once the item was administered, it was edited, and item analysis data was calculated and hand-entered on each card. The cards were then manually filed, ready to be edited and sorted for use on future tests.

This process was daunting by its very nature. Obtaining item analysis data required complex calculations that were tedious and time-consuming, even with the help of a calculator. Even when tests were electronically scored and data was provided by a computer program, each statistic still had to be hand-entered on the index cards. At test time, teachers had to hand-sort the items to meet the blueprint specifications and have the items re-typed for each new test. Another option was to photocopy the individual items to produce the test, which resulted in an unprofessional test appearance at best. In addition, this process required that the item analysis be re-calculated and entered on the index cards after each test administration.

While these procedures benefited the students of those enterprising teachers who undertook the arduous task of manually creating item banks, the effort required for developing and maintaining an up-to-date manual item bank required a nearly impossible time commitment for most teachers. As a result, the use of item banking for multiple-choice classroom testing was confined to those programs seriously committed to the concept and willing to devote the time to establishing a bank and, more importantly, to keeping it current. The software programs that are available today electronically manage the filing, sorting, storing, retrieval, and statistical calculation and updating of items for classroom testing, thereby freeing the teacher to commit the necessary time to ensuring the quality of the items in the bank.

Editing Items

While technology has the capacity for managing the administrative aspects of test development, the challenge for faculty is the quality enhancement of the items that comprise the bank. Quality is the most important issue in item banking; in fact, it is the central issue. The purpose of an item bank is to improve the items over time so that you eventually have a collection of high-quality items that will lighten the clerical burden of test construction and facilitate the development of reliable and valid classroom tests.

In order to have an item bank that is a viable force for improving the quality of classroom examinations, each item that is entered into the bank must be carefully edited. The first time an item is used in an exam there is no way to predict with any degree of certainty how the item will work, no matter how carefully it is constructed. The ambiguities and technical defects that were missed during test construction are revealed with item analysis and this information can be used to revise and improve the items for future use (Linn & Gronlund, 2000). The statistical data for each item that is an outcome of test administration is one of the most powerful tools available to teachers for improving test items. Considering the important role that tests play in education, it is essential that teachers use item analysis to improve the items they use in their classroom tests (Gullickson & Ellwein, 1985).

In addition to improving test items, item analysis also improves your item writing skills (Westwick, 1976). The more you analyze the actual statistical outcomes of test items, the more proficient you will become at recognizing the qualities that contribute to item difficulty and make them discriminate effectively. Practice with identifying defective items will help you to avoid flaws when you create items. Experience with rewording and modifying items based on item analysis will help you to develop expertise with writing original items and critiquing textbook item banks. The ultimate effect of experience with item analysis will be an improvement of your general test construction skills (Linn & Gronlund, 2000).

USING ITEM ANALYSIS   Chapter 10, "Interpreting Test Results," discusses how item analysis data can be used to analyze the functioning of an item so that decisions can be made about an overall test score. Item performance data is also a powerful vehicle for improving the reliability and validity of classroom tests by guiding the revision and improvement of the test items for inclusion in an item bank. General guidelines for using item analysis data include the following:

- Interpret the data with the size of the sample in mind. The larger the sample, the more dependable the data. Data for an item can be accumulated over time, which will increase the overall sample size. However, it is important to note that item analysis data refers to an item's performance on a particular test with a particular group. When the item is included with a different set of items to form a new test, or is used in the same test with a different group of students, the data is likely to change. Therefore, accumulated data gives you only a general picture of how an item is performing. Once you have your item bank established, however, you will find that many of the items perform consistently over time, particularly those that are edited based on item analysis data.

• Do not use item analysis data dogmatically. The data should be used as a guide for your professional judgment and expertise.

• The data associated with every option for an item must be analyzed. As the discussion of the quantitative test data analysis in Chapter 10, "Interpreting Test Results," points out, the p-value and the point biserial for an item correspond to the p-value and the point biserial for the item's correct answer. For example, note that in the sample item analysis data in Table 12.1, the p-value (0.68) and the point biserial (0.36) of the item correspond with the p-value (0.68) and the PBI (0.36) of choice B, the correct answer. These data give a picture of how well the item is working. However, it is also important to examine the analysis data for each of the distractors.

TABLE 12.1   Sample Item Analysis Data

Correct Answer = **B**
p-value (Difficulty): **0.68**
PBI (Point Biserial Index): **0.36**

Choice	Response Proportion	PBI
A	0.09	−0.08
B	**0.68**	**0.36**
C	0.12	−0.21
D	0.11	−0.25

• Consider every item for revision, but items that have a biserial of less than 0.20 should definitely be restructured. These items are not discriminating well between the high and low achievers on the test. Frequently, you will find that these items violate the guidelines for item writing. Examine the data for each option and rewrite the items, referring to the guidelines for stem and option construction that are presented in Chapter 6, "Developing Multiple-Choice Items."

• Determine the desirability of each item's difficulty level. When an item has a p-value of less than 0.30, it may be too difficult for the group. Similarly, an item that has a difficulty level of greater than 0.85 may be too easy for the group. It is not wise to set rigid parameters for retaining or eliminating an item; you should use your professional judgment to determine whether an item is appropriately difficult. Carefully review the actual item to determine whether the item difficulty level is desirable or if item revision is indicated.

- Distractors should be distracting. Every distractor should be selected; those that are not chosen by any test taker are not working as you planned. For example, if only the correct answer and one distractor are chosen for a four-option multiple-choice item, then the item is actually a two-option item. Options that are not selected are not contributing to the test and they probably should be revised.

- Look carefully at each option's biserial. An incorrect option that has a positive biserial or a correct option that has a negative biserial usually means that ambiguity in the stem or the options confused the students. If an item's correct option has a negative biserial and one or more distractors have a positive biserial, it means that the students who were the low achievers on the test selected the correct response more frequently than the students who were the high achievers on the test. This finding usually indicates that the high-achieving students were misled by item ambiguity or that the item is a trick item. It may also mean that all of the students were so confused by the item that they were guessing.

One situation that should raise a red flag occurs when an item's correct option has a positive biserial and one of the distractors also has a positive biserial. These results indicate that the distractors were confusing because they attracted the high-achieving students. These items require careful examination, both quantitatively and qualitatively, to determine whether to remove them from the test and how to revise them for future use.

The statistics obtained for each item provide information to guide you in improving the item. Remember that there are no dogmatic criteria for revising items; the data should be used as a guide in conjunction with your professional judgment. Item revision should be based on both qualitative and quantitative analyses of the item. Examine the items in Figures 12.1, 12.2, 12.3, 12.4, and 12.5. These examples illustrate how qualitative and quantitative analyses can be combined to improve your items for item banking.

These specific examples illustrate the potential of item analysis. The combination of statistical data and your professional expertise provides a powerful tool for test development that should not be overlooked.

INCORPORATING STUDENT COMMENTS The following examples illustrate that quantitative analysis cannot be used in isolation; your professional judgment is critical to successful item revision. Your qualitative review and the comments that accompany post-test review by both students and your colleagues provide a valuable resource for editing items before they are banked.

When revising items, it is most important to write distractors that attract the uninformed students. Student comments during test review often lend themselves to the creation of effective distractors. Be sure to take careful notes of student remarks during review sessions. These will provide you with valuable leads for developing effective distractors.

Selecting a Test Development Software Program

Test development/item banking software offers the most efficient means for streamlining the test development process. In fact, today's technology is so powerful that it cannot be ignored by anyone who is involved in the test development process. The

Original

A client has returned to her room from the recovery room S/P Billroth procedure. The nurse's initial assessment includes BP: 110/65, pulse 86 & regular, Resp. 18, Temp 100.8. Abdominal dressing dry and intact. Levin tube to low suction draining 25-30 cc/hr; yellow-brown drainage.

The nurse caring for the client notes the amount and color of the drainage from the Levin tube. The nurse concludes that the color indicates the presence of

A. normal gastric contents with residual bile.
B. normal gastric contents with old blood.
C. empty stomach with residual fecal matter.
D. empty stomach with residual gastric contents.

Correct Answer = **B**
p-value: **0.97**
PBI: **0.02**

Choice	Response Proportion	PBI
A	0.00	—
B	**0.97**	**0.02**
C	0.03	-0.02
D	0.00	—

Revised

A nurse assesses a client 24 hours after the client has had a Billroth procedure. The nurse's assessment includes: blood pressure, 110/65 mm Hg; pulse, 87/min and regular; respiration, 18/min; oral temperature, 100.0°F (37.8° C); nasogastric tube to low suction, draining 20-25 mL/hour of yellow-brown drainage. The nurse should recognize that these findings indicate

A. normal stomach contents with old blood.
B. impending hemorrhage from the stomach
C. reflux of intestinal contents with old blood
D. leakage of stomach contents into the peritoneum.

Correct Answer = **A**
p-value: **0.72**
PBI: **0.29**

Choice	Response Proportion	PBI
A	**0.72**	**0.29**
B	0.18	–0.09
C	0.07	–0.22
D	0.03	–0.23

The original item in this example violates several item-writing principles and the analysis data reflects the poor quality of the item. The stem is wordy, contains extraneous information, neglects to label vital signs, and is not grammatically consistent with options C or D. The item analysis indicates that the item was very easy, 97 percent of the students selected the correct answer. No one selected options A or D, and only three percent of the students chose option C, which indicates that these options should be revised. The item's point biserial is 0.02 which indicates that the item did not correlate well with the overall test. In short, this item is in need of major revision.

Item analysis for the revised item shows that the item's statistical results improved significantly. The revised example shortens the stem, labels the vital signs, and removes extraneous information. The revision also removes the distractors that did not work and substitutes more challenging distractors that relate to the stem. Option D in the revised item has the weakest results. You may decide to try the item again as it is, or edit option D for the next test. A distractor such as "presence of a low-grade surgical infection" may attract a greater number of the uninformed students. This example illustrates how item revision is an ongoing process that requires a combination of data and professional expertise.

FIGURE 12.1   Item analysis example #1

Original

A young man who has tumbled down a ski slope without one of his skis is lying at the foot of the slope complaining of severe pain in his lower leg. The nurse should

    A. elevate his injured leg.
    B. cover both legs with a blanket.
    C. assess for compartment syndrome.
    D. splint his injured leg.

Revised

A high school student falls down a flight of stairs at school and reports severe pain in the right lower leg. Which of these actions should a school nurse take?

    A. Splint the student's right leg.
    B. Elevate the student's right leg.
    C. Cover the student's right leg with a blanket.
    D. Assess the student's right leg for range of motion.

Correct Answer = **D**
p-value: **0.87**
PBI: **0.14**

Correct Answer = **A**
p-value: **0.71**
PBI: **0.37**

Choice	Response Proportion	PBI
A	0.08	-0.15
B	0.05	-0.05
C	0.00	—
D	**0.87**	**0.14**

Choice	Response Proportion	PBI
A	**0.71**	**0.37**
B	0.07	-0.20
C	0.03	-0.10
D	0.19	-0.48

This item illustrates an easy item; 87 percent of the students answered it correctly. The options in the original item are not homogeneous, which probably accounts for the poor biserial (0.14) for the question. While the correct answer has the only positive biserial (0.14) and two of the distractors have a negative biserial, option C was not chosen at all.

The revised item removes extraneous information, eliminates gender, increases the homogeneity of the options, and substitutes an alternative for option C. Note that the item analysis data indicates that the rewritten item was very effective. Because of the improvements, the revised item discriminates much more effectively than the original, the item is more difficult, every option was selected, and each of the distractors has a negative biserial.

FIGURE 12.2 Item analysis example #2

decision today is not whether to implement a test development software program; it is which program should you implement. In order to make an informed decision, you need to be aware of the capabilities offered by the available software programs and prioritize your needs to decide which options are most important for you.

Hardware Requirements

Your first concern is to identify your current hardware capabilities. It is essential that your computer system and electronic scanner are compatible with, and capable of

Original

The pharmacological action of antacids such as Mylanta is to

    A. coat the stomach mucosa.
    B. decrease gastric motility.
    C. elevate gastric pH.
    D. decrease duodenal pH.

Revised

A nurse should explain to a client that antacids, such as aluminum hydroxide (Mylanta), act to

    A. elevate gastric pH.
    B. coat the gastric mucosa.
    C. inhibit acid production.
    D. neutralize lactose intolerance.

Correct Answer = **C**
p-value: **0.56**
PBI: **0.24**

Correct answer = **A**
p-value: **0.67**
PBI: **0.43**

Choice	Response Proportion	PBI
A	0.44	-0.24
B	0.00	—
C	**0.56**	**0.24**
D	0.00	—

Choice	Response Proportion	PBI
A	**0.67**	**0.43**
B	0.10	-0.33
C	0.18	-0.26
D	0.04	-0.29

This item demonstrates how important it is to look at the whole picture. The item was difficult for the group, with a p-value of 0.56, and a reasonable point biserial (0.24). If your analysis stopped at this point, you would not see that options B and D were not chosen. You would miss the fact that the item is really a two-option item.

The revised item replaces both of the distractors that were not selected in the original item. It is evident from the statistical analysis that the revised item is a much more effective item. While it is still relatively difficult, it has an excellent point biserial, every option was selected, and all of the distractors have negative biserials. Option D was the weakest selection. This is a case where your professional judgment is needed to decide whether to revise the option or retest the item as it is to collect additional data.

FIGURE 12.3   Item analysis example #3

running, the program that you purchase. Your hardware capacity will limit your choice of software. On the other hand, if you are fortunate enough to have the funding to purchase a new computer and scanning system, you can select the software program of your dreams and purchase the hardware to suit the software.

Item Banking Facility

When reviewing software programs, it is important for you to identify what capability is essential for your particular needs, and then match those needs to a program that is

Original

Increasing the flow rate of total parenteral nutrition (TPN) above the prescribed rate is dangerous because it can result in

A. osmotic diuresis and hypo-glycemia.
B. hypoglycemia and dumping syndrome.
C. dumping syndrome and elec-trolyte imbalance.
D. electrolyte imbalance and osmotic diuresis.

Revised

A client is receiving total parenteral nutrition (TPN). A nurse should ensure that the TPN does not exceed the pre-scribed flow rate in order to prevent

A. hypoglycemia.
B. pneumothorax.
C. dumping syndrome.
D. electrolyte imbalance.

Correct Answer = **D**
p-value: **0.17**
PBI: **0.03**

Choice	Response Proportion	PBI
A	0.70	–0.13
B	0.11	0.17
C	0.03	–0.01
D	**0.17**	**0.03**

Correct Answer = **D**
p-value: **0.66**
PBI: **0.23**

Choice	Response Proportion	PBI
A	0.09	–0.23
B	0.09	–0.12
C	0.15	–0.10
D	**0.66**	**0.23**

With a p-value of 0.17 and a point biserial of 0.03, this item would definitely be a candidate for being discarded from the test. More than 70 percent of the students chose distractor A, which has a negative biserial (–0.13), while distractor B, which was chosen by almost 11 percent of the students, has a positive biserial (0.17). The difficulty level of the item and point biserial results indicate that the question is ambiguous, confusing, and in need of revision.

An examination of the item helps to explain the item analysis. This item violates item writing guidelines: Options A and C are partially correct, and all of the options overlap with at least one other option. This probably accounts for the students' confusion with the question. Should the item simply be discarded? If faculty think that the item is testing important information, it is worth an attempt at rewriting, especially since you can use the item analysis as a guide.

The rewrite of the item presented here simplifies the question while it still tests the key concept. The p-value of the revised item (0.66) keeps it in the difficult range. However, the item analysis shows that this version is much more effective than the original. The item has an acceptable point biserial, every option was selected, and every distractor has a negative biserial. Remember, every item should be considered for revision. Would you make any changes before reusing this item on a test?

FIGURE 12.4 Item analysis example #4

Original

Caring for a patient with a chest tube to pleur-evac system, the nurse knows that

A. bubbling in the water seal should be intermittent.
B. bubbling should be continuous and constant.
C. there should be no bubbling in the water seal.
D. bubbling will be seen in the suction regulator.

Revised

A client has a chest tube connected to an underwater-seal drainage system. Which of these observations of the drainage system should the nurse recognize as indicating that the system is functioning properly?

A. Fluctuations in the water-seal chamber.
B. Fluctuations in the collection chamber.
C. Continuous bubbling in the collection chamber.
D. Continuous bubbling in the water-seal chamber.

Correct Answer = **C**
p-value: **0.84**
PBI: **0.07**

Choice	Response Proportion	PBI
A	0.05	-0.16
B	0.11	0.03
C	**0.84**	**0.07**
D	0.00	—

Correct Answer = **A**
p-value: **0.78**
PBI: **0.30**

Choice	Response Proportion	PBI
A	**0.78**	**0.30**
B	0.05	-0.27
C	0.03	-0.02
D	0.12	-0.16

The item in Figure 12.5 has a p-value of 0.84 and a very weak biserial (0.07). One likely reason that the item was a poor discriminator is because distractor B has a positive biserial and no one chose distractor D. This is another item whose faults would be overlooked without careful item analysis.

The revision is composed of more homogeneous options that increased both the difficulty and discrimination values of the item. The revised item is more difficult than the original, many of the faults have been removed, and the item is no longer confusing the high-achieving students. All of the options are chosen and all distractors have negative biserials. Further revision of this item for retesting is a matter of professional judgment.

FIGURE 12.5 Item analysis example #5

as simple to operate as possible (Ward & Murray-Ward, 1994). Your initial review should seek to answer these questions:

- How many items can the bank hold?

- What item formats does the bank support?

- Is the manual clearly written and easy to understand?

- Is online support available?

- How is the security of the program maintained?

- What information can be included in a printout of the item bank?

Once you have this basic information, closely examine the features of the program, several of which are described in the discussion that follows. Take careful notes as you review each software program so that you will select the program that is best suited to your needs.

ITEM IMPORTING AND EXPORTING   This is an essential time-saving feature. If you have items stored in exams in electronic word processing files, or if you plan to use a commercially prepared item bank, you will want to make sure that the software program you purchase allows you to easily import these items into the item bank. If the program does not provide this function, you will have to key in the items manually. Carefully check this feature to make sure that the importing facility does not require complicated formatting of your current items. The most user-friendly programs allow you to simply save your word processing file as a .txt file, which is then automatically imported into an existing item bank. Once the items are in the bank they can be edited, revised, and coded.

Item importing is also important for future item development. As you are probably aware, only one person should work on an electronic file at one time. This is also true for item banking files. In order to avoid confusion and overwriting of the files when a course is taught by a group, one faculty member must be responsible for administering and maintaining the item bank files. Faculty in the group should be able to develop items in a word processing program, and the item banking program should have the capability of easily importing these items into the bank. A smooth importing facility allows faculty who do not have the test authoring software on their home computers to work on their items in a word processing program for importing into the item bank.

Exporting is another important feature. There are several reasons why you may want to export your items into a word processing file. Most importantly, you may decide to change software programs in the future. You do not want your items to be accessible only through the item bank. The export feature should be as seamless as the import feature. Make sure that you see a demonstration of both of these features before you purchase a software program.

WORD PROCESSING   Word processing capability is an essential feature that you should carefully consider. Because items will be constantly edited and revised over time, the word processing capability of the software program is very important. Features such as cutting, pasting, font selection, and spell checking are among the important features for word processing that help to streamline the item development process. Consider whether the program provides use of special characters and how it handles graphics. Some programs are not able to handle graphics in the item file; they must be kept in a separate file or even pasted into a hard copy of the test and photocopied. Make sure that the word processing capabilities are user friendly; an awkward program will become very frustrating over time and may interfere with continued faculty receptivity of the test development program.

ITEM CLASSIFICATION   In order to query an item bank to retrieve items, the items must be classified. The best scheme for organizing your banks is to have a bank for each course and classify the items in the course. Look for an item banking program that provides coding for at least eight to ten classification areas. A "drop down" box for entering codes is a valuable tool. This feature stores the codes and "drops them down" for you to mouse click so that you do not have to continually keyboard the codes into the program.

Determine the maximum number of classification areas you require. Suggestions for coding are shown in Table 12.2.

TABLE 12.2   Suggested item classification codes

• Nursing Process	• Topic
• Client Need	• Sub-topic
• Course Objective	• Key Words
• Learning Outcome	• Cognitive Level
• Content Area	• Author

In your efforts to develop a comprehensive coding plan, be careful that you do not make the scheme too complicated. Simplicity is best when you are beginning this process. The five categories in the first column in Table 12.2 are a good starting point. You can always add codes as your expertise develops. One word of caution: Although you can add codes, it can be very complicated to change codes, particularly on a large bank of items. Determining a classification scheme is another step in the test development process where planning is a crucial step.

Item codes allow you to query the bank to select items for inclusion on a test. For example, you could query the bank to see all of the items that have not yet been used this semester in a particular content area and objective. The program would allow you to view all of the items that meet those criteria. You could then select items from that group to meet the specific blueprint specifications for a test. Once the test is assembled, many programs will print a crossreference table or blueprint grid that specifies how many items are included on the test for each criteria.

When planning your classification scheme, it is important to be consistent across courses that may share item banks. The best approach is to obtain a consensus among the faculty for classification areas. You can leave one or two fields blank for use by an individual course or faculty member. Just consider the implications of having different fields if banks need to be combined or divided in the future.

SUPPLEMENTAL FIELDS   The item bank should have at least two supplemental fields for storing documentation information. When items are carefully documented, the validity of your tests is increased. Having fields such as item rationales and references readily accessible facilitates the process of editing and revising items. Most programs allow for these fields to be projected for group viewing. This facility is a great asset for student test review and also for faculty group review of items. Ease of availability encourages faculty to use these fields to increase the quality of their items. One advantage of having supplemental fields for each item is that the effort of documenting the item is never lost because the information in the field is permanently attached to the item. As Chapter 6, "Developing Multiple-Choice Items," suggests, items should be documented as they are written. Documenting old items can be a daunting task that should be approached gradually. Be realistic. If you set impossible goals, you will not succeed. The ultimate objective is to have a working item bank.

Test Assembly

Ease of test assembly is an important feature of test development software. Most programs provide for operator assembly or random selection of items by the computer, within query parameters defined by the teacher. When you initially use the software you will probably want to select the items from a hard copy, but you will soon find that selecting the items from the computer screen expedites the test assembly process. However, when a test contains items from several different teachers, it is usually preferable to have the teachers select their items from a hard copy of the item bank and have the bank administrator assemble the test on the computer.

Test assembly features vary among programs. Some allow on-screen viewing and selection of items; others require that you first select the items and then enter the item identification numbers into the program to assemble the test on the computer screen. Programs also vary in the number of variables that can be entered into a query for selecting items. In order to facilitate the selection of items to meet a test blueprint, choose a program that allows you to enter at least three categories (content area, objective, and date last used) into a query for item selection.

It is also wise to choose a program that allows you to print out a blueprint. This feature can also be used to generate cross-reference tables such as those illustrated in Figures 5.8, 5.9, and 5.10. The blueprint generated by the software is a precise picture of the criteria covered on the test, documenting content-related evidence of validity. Keep in mind that the more reports you want to generate, the more carefully your items must be coded and the more categories the software must allow you to include in a cross-reference.

Ward and Murray-Ward (1994) point out the desirability of several features for test-authoring software. These include the ability to perform the following:

- Produce an item map which indicates the key and the codes for each item on a test.

- Store and print general test directions.

- Automatically number pages and items.

- Print tests in a two-column format.

- Avoid inserting a page break in the middle of an item.

Additional features that enhance the quality of a software program include the ability to perform the following:

- Construct tests from multiple item banks.

- Indicate date-last-used for each item.

- Estimate the difficulty of the test based on the histories of the stored items.

- Create multiple versions of a test by scrambling items and/or options.

- Code items to prevent them from being scrambled.

- Code items that should not be included on the same exam.

- Print out a test blueprint or a cross-reference table.

Note that if the program has the ability to create multiple versions by scrambling items or item options, it is important that you are able to block an item from having its options scrambled. The options for certain items, such as those that have numerical answers, should be kept as they are written. Additionally, it frequently occurs that there are items that should not be included on the same test. The software should have the ability to code items so that items that cue each other are not used on the same exam.

Should you select a test-authoring program that allows you to develop and administer online tests? Most definitely. Should you purchase a program that is exclusively for online testing? Most definitely not, particularly if you are new to computerized test development. Whether you administer tests online or in a pencil and paper format, it is the quality of the items that matters most. Do not be misled by the bells and whistles of online testing programs. Online testing requires a very large bank of items, and it probably will take you several years before you can accumulate a large bank of quality items. In the meantime, it is important that you have the ability to administer pencil and paper tests so that you can generate that large bank of items.

However, when making your selection, remember that online test administration is becoming more prevalent. Even if you are using paper and pencil tests now, the capacity to deliver online tests should certainly be one factor in your selection of a test-authoring program. It makes sense to have the capability to administer tests online in the future no matter what your current capacity. Your goal with software selection should be to obtain the program that has the capabilities that you most want and need (Ward & Murray-Ward, 1994) to enable you to efficiently produce tests that are developed with high quality items.

Scoring and Reporting

Although tests that are administered online are automatically scored, printed tests require a separate scoring process, usually through an electronic scanning machine. Some programs require that you produce a key by hand, others score the test through the item bank where the correct answer is stored. When the need for a key is eliminated, the chance of error decreases, so a program that scores through the bank is preferable. Another essential feature for a scoring facility is the ability to adjust the scores based on post-test analysis.

A major concern when selecting a program is the type of score report produced by the program. The report should provide the test statistics that are included in Table 10.1. These statistics, as discussed in Chapter 10, "Interpreting Test Results," are essential for score interpretation. If the report does not include the item analysis data as illustrated in Figure 12.1, you will be handicapped in determining whether an item should be eliminated from a test, as well as with revising and improving your items.

In addition to creating reports for the teachers, many software programs provide individual student test reports. The report gives students individual feedback including the total test score and rationales for each item. When the report provides a printout of each student's individual item responses, the need to return answer sheets to the students during test review is eliminated. Some reports track the students' progress by providing them with their cumulative test average in a course.

Storage of Item Data History

Item analysis capability is an essential feature of a test-authoring software program. You cannot improve your items without the data on which to base your revisions. Some programs include a scoring and analysis program, while others interface with a separate analysis program. The important concern is that the item bank, scoring, and test analysis functions work smoothly together and that the item analysis data is electronically imported into the item bank. Manual entry of data is so tedious and time consuming that it eventually will be neglected. Therefore, electronic import and accumulation of analysis data are essential criteria when you are considering purchase of test-authoring software.

A software program should save an item's data analysis history including the p-value and point biserial for the items as well as for each distractor. Refer again to Table 12.1; it illustrates the minimum item data information that you should require of a test-authoring program. Look for a program that accumulates data in the item history. Accumulated data provides a much better estimate of how an item is working than the data results from a small sample. Important data, such as "date modified" and "date last used," is stored by some programs. "Date modified" is important when evaluating stored item analysis, and "date last used" is essential when assembling a test to ensure that items are not reused in the same semester and that they are rotated from year to year.

Gradebook Facility

Programs that do not have an internal gradebook usually have the ability to interface with an external gradebook program. These programs streamline the clerical aspects of tracking and calculating student grades. Exam scores are electronically entered into the grading program and course grades, based on the instructor input of grading criteria, are calculated and stored for each student.

Maintaining confidentiality when posting student grades is a serious concern for faculty. The ability to securely transmit grades to students is an important feature to obtain in a gradebook program. Some programs generate an anonymous identification number for each student and create a list for posting grades. Others have the ability to create an individual report for each student or transfer the grades to a secure Web site for student access.

Cost

Some may argue that cost should be your first concern. I think that a better approach is to look at several programs in various price ranges to provide you with a comprehensive basis for comparison so that you can carefully determine your needs and find a reasonable compromise between what you can afford and what you really want. When considering cost, remember to factor in the cost of new hardware if it is needed. Hardware includes your computer, monitor, printer, and scanner, and may also include a new copier. The ideal copier will collate and staple your exams. Sometimes, the cost of new hardware is money well spent; it actually could turn out to save you money. So, honestly assess your current hardware capabilities, and if you are severely limited by them, consider the feasibility of gradually purchasing new equipment.

An obvious cost concern is the price of the software. Examine the user agreements carefully. How many users are allowed to access the software? Are you purchasing or leasing the program? Will you be entitled to free upgrades? Is there a fee for technical support? All of these issues will affect the ultimate cost of the program.

There are also hidden costs associated with computerized test administration. How expensive are the scannable sheets that are required for the program? Will you need to hire additional staff to maintain the bank? Will word processors be needed to key in current questions? Computerized test development software is a longterm cost saver. However, you need to take a close look at your start-up costs so that you do not derail your project before it is begun.

Carefully consider each of the questions in Figure 12.6 before you purchase a test development software program.

Implementing Test Development Software

Planning is the most important step for developing an item bank (Rudner, 1998). In order to ensure that your decision to institute electronic test development will be actualized, a team of committed individuals must take the initiative to generate a plan of action that will lay the groundwork for successful implementation of the software. When developing the plan, it is crucial to acknowledge that purchase and application of test development software is not an end in itself; the software is a tool that is only as good as the information it manipulates. The axiom "garbage in, garbage out," applies here. The critical first step is to follow the guidelines presented in this book to formulate a plan for the systematic assessment of learning outcomes across the curriculum. Then you can evaluate the available software to determine which program will best facilitate the ongoing implementation of your systematic assessment plan.

You may have the impression from the discussion in the previous section that test development software is extremely complex. If you think about it, you will probably agree that this is a typical reaction to first exposure to any new software program, particularly when you are reading about it without having the program to manipulate. Working in the actual program will give you a much better feel for how it operates. Be

What are your hardware capabilities?

How is the security of the program maintained?

How many items can the bank hold?

What information can be included in a printout of the item bank?

What item formats does the bank support?

Is the manual clearly written and easy to understand?

Is online support available?

Is there a charge for technical support?

How does the program import and export items?

Are you satisfied with the demonstration of the import and export functions?

Does the word processing program provide easy access to these features?
- Spell checking
- Font selection
- Cutting and pasting

Does the number of classification areas meet your needs?

Does the program have drop-down boxes to facilitate item classification?

Does the number of supplemental fields meet your needs?

Does the program print a cross reference table for the test?

Examine the case in which the program asssembles a test:

How many classification areas can be entered in a query for selecting items for a test?

What is the procedure for entering test specifications into the program, on screen and/or hard copy?

Can the software create a test based on the test blueprint?

Does the test assembly have the capacity to access more than one bank?

Can the user view items by user-specified criteria?

Can more than one version of the test be created?

If item options can be scrambled, can an item be coded to prevent scrambling of its options?

Can items that should not be used together on an exam be coded?

Does the test developer function estimate the difficulty of the test based on stored item histories?

Does the software have these features?
- Produces print copies of test
- Administers tests online
- Maps items with keys and codes
- Stores and prints test direction
- Automatically numbers pages
- Has the ability to print tests in one- or two-column format

FIGURE 12.6   Questions to ask when assessing test development software (*continues*)

(continued)

How are the tests scored, both online and pencil and paper?

Does a key need to be manually entered?

What is the availability and cost of required scannable forms?

How does the program adjust the scores based on post-test analysis?

Examine the adequacy of the score report:

What test statistics are included in the test analysis?

What statistical data is included in the individual item analysis?

What item data is automatically stored in the item history?

Is the item data accumulated in the item history?

Is date-last-used and date-last-edited stored with the item?

If a student report is available, what information does it provide?

Does the program have, or interface with, a gradebook program?

How user-friendly are the gradebook functions?

How flexible is the input of the grading criteria?

Does the gradebook keep running calculations of each student's grades?

How does the gradebook facilitate the posting of student grades?

What is the cost of hardware replacement or upgrade?

What does the software cost?

Are current customers entitled to discounted upgrades?

Have you looked for hidden costs associated with computerized testing?

FIGURE 12.6   Questions to ask when assessing test development software

sure to obtain demo disks for each of the programs that you want to evaluate. It is important that the program you purchase be user-friendly, because the faculty who will use the program will have a wide range of computer ability.

Appointing Test Bank Administrators

Once you have developed your plan, purchased your software, and created your item classification scheme, you are ready to employ the software to create your item bank. At this point, it is essential that one or more item bank administrators be appointed if they are not already in place. While item banking software streamlines the process of test development, it is a complex process that involves a wide cast of participants. When everyone is in charge, no one is in charge. Successful implementation of an item bank requires management and coordination.

The responsibility for making the decision for how to manage the program lies with the faculty as a group. A variety of factors will enter into the decision, including: whether courses are taught by a group or individual faculty, the size of the program, the number of faculty members, the computer expertise of the faculty, the availability of technical support on the campus, and the willingness of faculty to participate as coordinators of the item bank. Administering an item bank, especially when it is being developed, is a sizable responsibility that requires well-organized individuals who have at least basic computer skills, and are willing to devote the time and face the challenges of implementing change. A practical approach is to assign one bank administrator for each course, with these administrators forming the item bank committee that oversees the entire bank. Some programs choose to use the services of a consultant to facilitate the initiation of the bank. Although this approach is expensive initially, a consultant who is experienced at setting up test development software for a nursing program will save you time, and could save you money, in the long run.

Faculty who commit to instituting and administering the item bank are making a very worthwhile contribution to the quality of student education. Directing the operation of an item bank should not be considered an "extra" assignment. It is a time-consuming responsibility, particularly during the initiation of the bank that should be acknowledged in terms of faculty workload. This may be a hard sell to school administration, but the burden of this responsibility could easily overwhelm faculty volunteers if they are expected to carry a full workload in addition to item banking coordination. Considering item bank administration as part of a faculty member's workload ensures that the faculty who volunteer to administer the bank will be able to devote the necessary time to ensure the successful implementation of the software.

The work of the faculty administrators can be greatly facilitated if a member of the support staff develops expertise in managing the clerical aspects of the item bank. Duties such as scanning, entering rosters, importing and exporting items, importing item data, printing hard copies of tests and item banks, and even assembling tests based on faculty selection are responsibilities that can be assumed by a knowledgeable support staff member under the direction of the bank administrator. Do not be misled into believing that clerical staff can assume sole responsibility for the item bank. Remember, the biggest concern with item banking is the quality of the questions. Coding, item editing, and interpreting item analysis are among the roles of the administrator that can be assumed only by a faculty member.

Establishing Procedures

In order to expedite item banking, implementation procedures must be established to direct the process. It is very important that the entire faculty take ownership of the item bank. Therefore, although the bank administrators may draft the procedures, the entire faculty should have input into making the final decision for the processes that direct the item bank. Consult with other schools who are using the software. Keep the procedures as simple as possible and have written guidelines to avoid confusion. Remember, your plan does not have to be perfect: Keep it flexible and open to change as your test development process evolves.

ITEM EDITING AND REVISION   Testing companies subject their items to rigorous review by content experts and, in addition, they employ a professional editor to ensure that the items on their tests adhere to their style guides. While schools cannot be held to these standards, it is important that a system be developed to edit and revise all items based on both content and the style guide before they are entered into the bank.

Every item that is proposed for bank entry should be subjected to the same process. This is a task that is very time consuming when a bank is initiated, but it becomes more manageable once the bank is established. The process can be handled by the individual bank administrators or by the item bank committee. Whichever system is employed, it is essential that an edited item be returned to the faculty author for final approval before it is entered into the bank.

SELECTING EXAM ITEMS   The procedure for selecting items for inclusion in a test will be largely determined by the software program that you select. However, you will have to set up a logistical plan. In order to create a test from a software bank, all of the test items must be in the bank. If you have established a process for entering items into the bank, all of the items in the bank will meet the faculty's standards for item quality. Therefore, junior faculty or adjunct instructors could use the bank and be assured of the quality of the items that they select for a test.

While having an item bank improves item quality, it is essential that faculty have the freedom and ability to compose new items. In fact, faculty item-writing efforts should be encouraged because the larger the bank, the more useful it will be. All items should go through the same process for entry into the bank. One very important note: Editing is always easier than writing the original. The item-editing process should be a helpful and congenial one.

If exams are composed by one person, the selection process is simple. The faculty member can choose items to meet the blueprint from either a hard copy of the bank or on the computer screen. When a faculty group is involved in the selection process, it is usually best to provide each with the test blueprint and a hard copy of the items that relate to their piece of the course. Make sure that the hard copy includes the stored difficulty and discrimination values, the classifications, and the date last used for each item. This information will assist faculty in selecting items and will ensure that items are not reused in a semester. In fact, if your bank is large enough, it is wise to use as few of the same items as possible in consecutive years.

Once the items are selected, the bank administrator should collect the selections of each faculty and assemble the exam as discussed in Chapter 8, "Assembling, Administering, and Scoring a Test." During pre-test review, each faculty member should ensure that their item selections have been accurately entered on the test.

POST-TEST ITEM REVISION   The first section of this chapter addresses the procedure for post-test item revision. When the item data is automatically entered into the item bank, item revision is facilitated. Your task is to determine how to implement the revision. The bank administrator, the item bank committee, or the faculty author of the item can make revisions. When you are new to this process it is probably best to work on revisions as a group, or circulate hard copies of the items for faculty input. It is essential that you do not overlook this step in the test development process. Item revision based on analysis data is the key to quality test items. Maintaining a system will ensure that revision does not get put off and eventually forgotten.

Figure 12.7 is an example of an item bank screen. Note that it includes fields for all of the requirements identified for quality test development software. Solution, reference, classification, item analysis data, date last used, and date modified are all available to facilitate test development, item analysis, and item revision.

Refer to Figure 12.8 for a summary of the steps for implementing a test development software program.

Cardiovascular 101

A client who is receiving intravenous heparin has an activated thromboplastin time (APTT) of two and one-half times the control. In addition to documenting the finding, which of these actions would be appropriate for a nurse to take?

A. Call the lab for a stat repeat of the test.

B. Discontinue the client's heparin infusion immediately.

C. Continue to monitor the client.*

D. Alert the blood bank to have a unit of packed cells available.

Solution

This question asks the student to recognize that the APTT should be between 1.5 and 2.5 times the control for a client who is receiving heparin. It requires the student to apply that information. In this question, while the client's APTT is within the range, it is at the top of the range. The nurse could also check the client's vital signs, or observe for adverse effects, such as hematuria. However, the question asks the student to discriminate among the options offered, and only one of these is correct.

Reference

Shannon, M. T., & Wilson, B. A. (1992). *Govoni & Hayes: Drugs and Nursing Implications.* Norwalk, CT: Appleton and Lange, p. 645.

Nsg Process	Client Need	Objective*	L Outcome*	Content	Cog Level	Author
Implement	Pharm therapy	Crit Think/3	3/11	Anticoag.	App	Smith

Cumulative Item Analysis

p(Diff) value	PBI
0.74	0.65

Response Frequencies (%)

A	B	C	D	E
13	3	10	74	NA

Date Last Used	Date Modified
11/12/2001	12/2/2000

*Objectives and Learning Outcomes are assigned a number to facilitate entry into classification scheme.

FIGURE 12.7   Sample item bank screen

- Assemble a team of committed faculty members

- Develop plan for systematic assessment of outcomes

- Review and select test development software

- Create item classification scheme

- Appoint item bank administrators

- Establish process for item editing, revision, and inclusion in bank

- Establish procedure for selecting items for exams

- Determine procedure for revising items based on post-test analysis

FIGURE 12.8   Implementing test development software

Incorporating Textbook Item Banks

Most current nursing textbooks provide faculty with a test bank of items that complement the text. Do not assume that these items are of high quality simply because they have been published. In fact, the quality of these banks varies widely. Very few banks contain items that have been pilot-tested on students, so there are no assurances that these items will function well on a test.

While textbook items can be helpful, they must be subjected to the same rigorous standards that you require of your own items, which means that most of them require revision. Examine the items carefully. In many cases, the concept being tested is worthwhile, but the item is not constructed in accordance with the guidelines presented in Chapter 6, "Developing Multiple-Choice Test Items," and Chapter 7, "Writing Critical Thinking Multiple-Choice Test Items." Most often, the distractors need work. Take advantage of these banks as a valuable resource for finding items to revise and incorporate into your item bank.

Figure 12.9 identifies several Web sites where more information about specific test development software programs can be found.

Summary

While test-authoring software provides faculty with an invaluable tool for facilitating the test development process, it can fulfill its potential only if it is part of a carefully developed plan for systematic assessment. As with all technology, the quality of the final product is related to the human input. Before you can successfully use a testing software program to implement an overall assessment plan, you must be conversant with the principles of assessment.

Item analysis data is a valuable tool that is provided by test development software. The data provided for each item must be combined with your professional expertise to enhance the quality of your test items. General guidelines and specific examples are

www.assess.com

www.atrixware.com

www.catinc.com

www.chariot.com

www.escoinst.com

www.lxrtest.com

www.questionmark.com

www.scantron.com

www.softwarefornurses.com

FIGURE 12.9 Web sites for test development software information

combined in this chapter to provide faculty with direction for implementing test revision based on item analysis.

Having a clear idea of your assessment needs is a prerequisite for making an informed decision about which software program to purchase. A wide variety of programs are currently available, providing item banking and test development capabilities with the capacity for online test administration. Making your selection will undoubtedly require that you make some compromises, but the potential of test development software requires that you make a decision. There is no reason to put off your purchase. The software that is available is fully capable of handling the needs of a school-based testing program. Consult with your colleagues, contact schools that are successfully using the software, follow the guidelines provided in this chapter to make a decision, and take the initiative to move your assessment program into the 21st century. The longer you wait, the more time is wasted.

A Basic Test Statistics

MEASURES OF CENTRAL TENDENCY	Measures designed to provide a single value that best represents the typical score in a distribution.

Mean — The score that represents the arithmetic average on a test. Obtained by dividing the sum of a set of scores by the number of scores.

Median — The middle score in a set of ranked scores that divides the group into two equal halves (the 50th percentile).

Mode — The score that occurs most frequently in a set of scores.

PERCENTILE RANK — A score that indicates the percentage of lower scores in the norm group. If a score of 54 on a test is equal to the 40th percentile, it indicates that 40 percent of the students in the group achieved a score equal to or lower than 54 while 60 percent of those in the group received scores higher than 54. A percentile does not show what percent of questions the examinee answered correctly on the test.

CORRELATION COEFFICIENT — An index that indicates the relationship between two sets of measures. This index ranges from –1.0, which indicates a perfect negative relationship, to + 1.0, which indicates a perfect positive relationship. A value of 0.0 indicates that there is no relationship between the two measures.

RELIABILITY COEFFICIENT	An index of the consistency of test scores. This index ranges from 1.0, which is perfect consistency, to 0.0, which indicates the absence of reliability.
VARIANCE (SD^2) and STANDARD DEVIATION (SD)	A measure of the dispersion of scores around the mean of a distribution. The more the scores cluster around the mean, the smaller the variance. The smaller the variance (SD^2), the greater the similarity of the group. SD is the square root of the variance. Large values of these indices indicate that the scores are spread out away from the mean.
STANDARD ERROR OF MEASUREMENT (SEM)	An estimate of the possible amount by which a score (or group of scores) can differ from the true score, based on errors in measurement. The larger the SEM, the less reliable the score.
DIFFICULTY INDEX (p-value)	The percent of correct responses to an item. This value is obtained by dividing the sum of those who answered the item correctly by the total number who took the test. This index ranges from 0.0 to +1.0, with 0.0 indicating that no one answered correctly and +1.0 indicating that all test takers answered the item correctly.
DISCRIMINATION INDEX (D value) or POINT-BISERIAL INDEX (PBI)	Indicates the quality of a test item by identifying the capability of the item to differentiate between high scorers and low scorers on a test. The higher the D value or PBI, the better the test item. The index ranges between –1.0 and +1.0. A positive discrimination index occurs when more students in the highest-scoring group answered the item correctly than those in the lowest-scoring group. A negative index means that more students in the lowest-scoring group answered the item correctly than those in the highest-scoring group.

B Basic Style Guide

This guide is a brief outline of the rules that apply to item writing. The rules of grammar and punctuation are very complex, so you should have at least one good style reference if you write at all. Each of the references cited at the end of this appendix is worth owning. Remember, no document is read more carefully than your tests are by the students who take them.

- Write all items in the present tense. Keeping all sentences in the present tense avoids confusion concerning the time of different actions and makes the problem in the question seem to be occurring as the student is attempting to solve it:

  > A nurse is assessing a client . . .
  >
  > NOT
  >
  > A nurse assessed a client . . .

- Avoid using the passive voice in an item. The active voice means that the subject of the sentence is the doer. The subject is acted upon in the passive voice. The active voice is more direct and concise than the passive voice. Misuse of voice does not constitute a grammatical error, but it does affect the readability of the items:

  > A nurse is assessing a client.
  >
  > NOT
  >
  > The client is being assessed by a nurse.

- End a stem that presents a question with a question mark (?), followed by options that are complete sentences. Begin each option with an upper-case letter, and end it with a period:

  > Which of these actions should a nurse take?
  >
  > A. Obtain the client's blood pressure.
  > B. Elevate the head of the client's bed.
  > C. Give the client the prescribed sedative.
  > D. Instruct the client to cough and take deep breaths.

- Do not punctuate at the end of a stem that is an incomplete statement. Begin each option that is completing the stem with a lower-case letter, and end the option with a period:

    A nurse should assess the client for

    A. hyperthermia.

    B. rusty sputum.

    C. chest pain.

    D. hypotension.

- Use "nurse" instead of "you" as the subject of the question:

    Which of these questions should a nurse ask?

    NOT

    Which of these questions should you ask?

- Use "should" instead of "would." *Should* denotes obligation or necessity, while *would* suggests what might happen. Items should focus on what should occur, not what an individual nurse might do. Technically, because anything might happen, every option that follows the word *would* might be correct:

    Which of these measures should a nurse include in the client's care plan?

    NOT

    Which of these measures would a nurse include in the client's care plan?

- Be consistent with terms. Decide on options such as client or patient, prescription or order, and physician or doctor and use them consistently. Client is the preferred term in most textbooks and on the licensure and certification exams.

    Which of these instructions should a nurse give to a client?

- Be careful with the use of "signs" and "symptoms." A sign is an objective finding that is observed by an examiner. A symptom is a subjective indication as perceived by the client. A manifestation is a perceptible indication of a disease. If "sign" is used in the stem, every option that follows must be a "sign." If "symptom" is used, every option that follows must be a "symptom." Use "manifestation" if the options include both signs and symptoms.

    A nurse should observe the client for which of these manifestations?

- "A" is the indefinite article that refers to a person who is not previously specified. "The" is an adjective that is used before a person who has already been mentioned. The first time you refer to a nurse or a client, use "a." The second time, use "the":

    A nurse is teaching a client who is on a low sodium diet. Which of these instructions should the nurse give to the client?

- Avoid ambiguities by specifying who is saying or doing what to whom in the stem. Do not leave anything to the imagination of the examinees:

  > Which of these statements, if made by a client who is on a low sodium diet, should indicate to a nurse that the client is adhering to the diet prescription?
  > NOT
  > Which of these statements should indicate to a nurse that a client understands how to follow a low sodium diet? (It is unclear who is making the statement.)

- Avoid using descriptors for clients or nurses. Gender, names, ages, marital status, and occupation are all extraneous information that could introduce bias into your item unless these descriptors pertain to the problem that is being posed:

  > A nurse is caring for a client who has had an appendectomy . . .
  > NOT
  > A nurse is caring for Mrs. Bock, a 45-year-old woman who has had an appendectomy . . .

- Health problems are very unflattering adjectives. Use the following:

  > A client who has hypertension
  > NOT
  > A hypertensive client

- Use the term "medication" for all legal medications. Save the term "drug" for reference to illegal substances:

  > A client is taking all of these medications.
  > NOT
  > A client is taking all of these drugs.

- Refer to all medications with both the generic and trade name the first time they appear in a stem. The second reference can use either name:

  > A client is taking furosemide (Lasix). Which of these side effects of Lasix should a nurse caution the client about?

- Clarify all abbreviations. For example, decide whether to use mL or ml, and use them consistently. Periods are not necessary after an abbreviation. Use abbreviations only after a number.

  > How many milliliters should the client receive?
  > NOT
  > How many mL should the client receive?

- The first time a phrase that is commonly referred to as an abbreviation is used, spell out the phrase and put the abbreviation in parentheses (no matter how common you think the abbreviation is). Use only the abbreviation once it is introduced:

    A client is scheduled to have a nasogastric tube (NGT) inserted. Which of these explanations should a nurse offer the client about the purpose of the NGT?

- Label all laboratory values and vital signs:

    A client has a blood pressure of 110/82 mm Hg and serum potassium of 3.8 mEq/L.

    NOT

    A client has a blood pressure of 110/82 and serum potassium of 3.8.

- Use both Fahrenheit and Centigrade when reporting temperature:

    A client has a temperature of 100.4°F (98°C).

    NOT

    A client has a temperature of 100.4° F.

    or WORSE

    A client has a temperature of 100.4°.

- A "complaining" client has a very negative connotation. Use "reports" instead:

    A client reports having abdominal pain.

    NOT

    A client complains of abdominal pain.

- Avoid referring to a client as being "with" a health problem. "With" is a preposition that means "in the company of," or "having as a possession, attribute, or feature." A client is not accompanied by a health problem and certainly would not consider a health problem to be an attribute or a characteristic. "Has" is the third-person, present singular of the verb "have." One meaning of have is "to be affected by something, particularly something of a medical nature." Use a client "who has" a health problem:

    A client who has colon cancer . . .

    NOT

    A client with colon cancer . . .

- In order to avoid labeling a client who is diagnosed with a mental illness, it is more acceptable to refer to the client as being "diagnosed with" than to say a client "who has" a mental illness:

    A client who has a diagnosis of bipolar disorder . . .

    NOT

A client who has bipolar disorder . . .

> or WORSE

A client with bipolar disorder . . .

- It is inappropriate to use contractions in formal writing, and a test should be considered formal. It is acceptable to use contractions when you are quoting someone:

  A nurse who **cannot** understand what a client is saying says to the client, "Could you repeat what you just said. I didn't understand you."

  > NOT

  A nurse who **can't** understand what a client is saying says to the client, "I didn't understand you. Could you repeat what you just said?"

- Avoid using brand names that might be unfamiliar to some students:

  A new mother says to a nurse, "My baby just finished drinking the infant formula . . . "

  > NOT

  A new mother says to a nurse, "My baby just finished drinking the Enfamil . . . "

- A measure is an action that is a means to an end. The activities related to the planning phase of the nursing process are ongoing series of actions that are designed to achieve a planned outcome. The use of a verb here would connote that the action will occur only once instead of ongoing until the outcome is achieved. Express measures that connote ongoing activities as gerunds. A gerund is a verb plus -*ing* that acts as a noun:

  Which of these measures should a nurse include in the care plan for a client who has a nursing diagnosis of fluid volume deficit?

  A. Monitoring . . .

  B. Observing . . .

  C. Measuring . . .

  D. Providing . . .

  > NOT

  A. Monitor . . .

  B. Observe . . .

  C. Measure . . .

  D. Provide . . .

- Use a verb for an activity that occurs as a one-time action. These actions relate to the implementation phase of the nursing process.

    Which of these actions should a nurse take when a client develops dyspnea?

    A. Stop . . .

    B. Elevate . . .

    C. Report . . .

    D. Administer . . .

    NOT

    A. Stopping . . .

    B. Elevating . . .

    C. Reporting . . .

    D. Administering . . .

- Spell out numbers one through nine; write numbers 10 and higher as figures. This rule does not apply to ages, figures containing decimals, percentages, temperature, dates, math calculations, or times of day, however:

    A client who has exercised for eight minutes . . .

    A 6-year-old child . . .

    A client who has been in surgery for 16 hours . . .

- Arrange numbers in options in sequence, usually from smallest to largest. Scrambled values require students to hunt for the answer:

    A. 11

    B. 16

    C. 32

    D. 46

    NOT

    A. 32

    B. 46

    C. 11

    D. 16

- Terms should also be arranged in sequence:

    A nurse should identify the client's anxiety level as

    A. mild.

    B. moderate.

    C. severe.

    D. panic.

NOT

A nurse should identify the client's anxiety level as

    A. severe.

    B. panic.

    C. mild.

    D. moderate.

- Make the style agree in a series that includes numbers that would ordinarily be spelled out and numbers that would ordinarily be given as figures:

    A. 2

    B. 6

    C. 14

    D. 19

    NOT

    A. Two

    B. Six

    C. 14

    D. 19

- Spell out a number that begins a sentence:

    Twenty minutes after taking a medication . . .

    NOT

    20 minutes after taking a medication . . .

- Omit the period after a number in an option. It could be misconstrued as a decimal point and could cause confusion:

    A. 9

    B. 12

    C. 16

    D. 22

    NOT

    A. 9.

    B. 16.

    C. 22.

    D. 12.

- When the stem contains a word that reverses the meaning of the question, the font for the negative word should be bold, italic, and small caps in order to draw attention to the reversal. Highlight only words that reverse the meaning of the stem. Once you start to highlight adjectives and adverbs, such as first, last, most, least, and priority, the impact of highlighting diminishes. Students are more likely to overlook the emphasis placed upon the word.

> Which of these statements, if made by the client, should indicate to a nurse that the client needs FURTHER instruction?
>
> NOT
>
> Which of these statements, if made by the client, should indicate to a nurse that the client needs further instruction?

- Use hyphens when two or more adjectives are placed together to modify a noun:

> A 2-year-old child . . .
>
> A nurse uses a one-inch needle . . .
>
> A well-known celebrity is admitted . . .

Remember, the key word in the phrase "style guide" is **guide**. All of these suggestions are guidelines. Some of the guidelines are designed to raise a red flag—to alert you to a potential problem with an item and to caution you to closely examine the language you have used. When considering these guidelines, keep in mind that these style guides are associated with items that work successfully on multiple-choice exams. In the end, you are the final judge of the appropriateness of an item.

References

Jordan L. (Ed.). (1976). *The New York Times: Manual of style and usage.* New York: The New York Times.

Stilman A. (1997). *Grammatically correct: The writer's essential guide.* Cincinnati: F & W Publications.

Strunk W and White E B. (2000). *The elements of style.* (4th ed.). Boston: Allyn and Bacon.

C Targeting Cognitive Levels for Item Writing

KNOWLEDGE: Recalling material that was previously learned. Refers to the simple remembering of a fact, concept, theory, or principle. The learner is expected to recall information exactly as presented in a textbook or from a classroom lecture and then select the correct answer from the choices presented. Knowledge questions do **not** require understanding or judgment. Knowledge questions test the student's ability to remember previously learned facts, to recall information, and to recognize the correct choice.

KNOWLEDGE VERBS:

Define	Recognize
Identify	Relate
Know	Reproduce
List	Select
Name	State
Quote	Tell
Recall	Write

SAMPLE ITEM:

A nurse should tell a client who has hypothyroidism that the purpose of levothyroxine (Synthroid) is to

    A. replace thyroid hormone.*

    B. stimulate the action of the thyroid gland.

    C. provide thyroid-stimulating hormone.

    D. block the stimulation of the thyroid gland.

COMPREHENSION: The ability to grasp the meaning of material that is shown by translating material from one form to another. Comprehension questions test the student's ability to understand information, translate facts, interpret the importance of the information, take in information and "give it back" another way, and make predictions based on understanding.

COMPREHENSION VERBS:

Change	Infer
Compare	Interpret
Convert	Outline
Describe	Rank
Differentiate	Rearrange
Discuss	Reorder
Distinguish	Rephrase
Estimate	Reword
Explain	Summarize
Extrapolate	Translate
Illustrate	Transform

SAMPLE ITEM:

A nurse should explain to a client who is taking wafarin sodium (Coumadin) the need to limit the intake of which of these foods?

    A. Liver

    B. Spinach*

    C. Whole milk

    D. Grapefruit

APPLICATION: The ability to use learned material in new and concrete situations. Application questions test the student's ability to apply concepts, laws, methods, phenomena, principles, procedures, rules, theories, and to solve problems in unique, real-life situations.

APPLICATION VERBS:

Accelerate	Elevate	Offer
Ascertain	Employ	Operate
Ask	Encourage	Prevent
Apply	Enhance	Prepare
Arrange	Ensure	Promote
Assist	Examine	Relate
Associate	Formulate	Remove
Avoid	Generalize	Restrict
Balance	Guide	Revise
Calculate	Identify	Schedule
Check	Illustrate	Show
Classify	Initiate	Solve
Compute	Instruct	Stop
Compose	Limit	Suppress
Construct	Locate	Teach
Control	Measure	Test
Design	Minimize	Transfer
Develop	Modify	Use
Demonstrate	Motivate	Utilize
Determine	Obtain	
Discourage	Observe	

SAMPLE ITEM:

A client who is taking NPH insulin (Humulin N) every morning reports feeling weak and tremulous in the mid-afternoon. Which of these actions should a nurse initiate?

    A. Take the client's blood pressure.

    B. Give the client's PRN dose of insulin.

    C. Check the client's capillary blood sugar.*

    D. Advise the client to lie down with legs elevated.

ANALYSIS: The ability to break down material into its component parts so that its organizational structure can be understood. Analysis questions test the student's ability to break down information, to see a relationship among the parts, to recognize the effects, and to understand the meaning of information.

ANALYSIS VERBS:

Analyze	Divide
Associate	Estimate
Categorize	Examine
Compare	Infer
Contrast	Investigate
Correlate	Look for trends
Delineate	Order
Deduce	Question
Detect	Recognize error
Determine	Separate
Differentiate	Solve
Diagram	Subdivide
Distinguish	Verify

SAMPLE ITEM:

Which of these manifestations, if identified in a client during the immediate postoperative period, should a nurse associate with the development of hypovolemic shock?

A. Hypertension

B. Increased pulse*

C. Hyperthermia

D. Rapid capillary refill

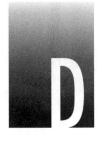

D Sample Item Stems for Phases of the Nursing Process

I. ASSESSMENT
Process of collecting, verifying and communicating relevant client data

Which of these (manifestations, side effects) should a nurse investigate first when assessing a client who has (undergone a dx test, nursing dx, medical dx, medication prescription)?

A nurse assesses that a client who has (dx) has (manifestations, vital signs). What additional data should the nurse collect to establish a nursing diagnosis of (. . .)? What (information, data) should the nurse obtain first?

When assessing a client who has (dx), a nurse should determine whether the client has which of these (signs, symptoms, clinical manifestations, lab values)?

Which of these questions would be the most important for a nurse to ask a client who has (dx, manifestations)?

In order to identify whether a client is developing a (side effect of medication, complication of a procedure, progression of a disease), which of these questions should a nurse ask the client? Which of these assessments should a nurse make?

Which of these questions would be the most appropriate for a nurse to ask a client to assist in establishing a nursing diagnosis of . . . ?

Which of these data would be most important for a nurse to obtain when assessing a client who has (manifestation, dx)?

A nurse assesses that a client who has (dx) has (manifestation). What further information should the nurse obtain? Which of these questions would be the most important for the nurse to ask the client?

A client who has (dx) develops (manifestations, vital signs). What additional data should a nurse obtain?

A nurse assesses that a client has all of these (manifestations, vital signs). Which one is most likely related to (dx)?

II. ANALYSIS

Process of interpreting assessment data to identify actual or potential client health problems

A nurse identifies that a client who has (dx) demonstrates (manifestations, lab values). This finding would help substantiate a nursing diagnosis of . . .

A client who has (dx) says to a nurse, " . . . " A nurse should recognize this statement as indicative of . . .

When assessing a client who has (dx), which of these finding would indicate (complication, advanced disease progress)?

Which of these factors in a client's history is most likely related to the development of (dx)?

A nurse assesses that a client who has (dx) has a (laboratory test, dx test) that reveals . . . Which of these nursing diagnoses should receive priority for this client?

A nurse assesses that a client who has (dx) has a (laboratory test, dx test) that reveals . . . . Which of these nursing diagnoses is appropriate for this client?

Which of these findings, if identified in a client who (has dx, had procedure, is taking medication), should a nurse report to a physician immediately?

A nurse assesses a client who (has dx) (is taking medication). Which of these client findings would require immediate follow up by the nurse?

A nurse obtains a health history from a client who (has dx) (is taking medication). Which of these client findings should the nurse follow up immediately?

Which of these findings, if identified in a client who (has dx, is receiving rx), would indicate that the client is at risk for developing (complication)?

A nurse should recognize that a client who (has dx) (is taking medication) is at risk for developing (complication, side effect) if the client . . .

A client who has (dx, been in an accident, sustained an injury) is admitted to the emergency department with (several manifestations). Which of the injuries should be treated first?

III. PLANNING

Process of establishing desired client outcomes and designing strategies to achieve those outcomes

Which of these outcomes would be most appropriate for a nurse to establish with a client who has a (nursing dx, medical dx) of . . . ?

A nurse is developing a plan of care with a client who has (nursing dx, medical dx). Which of these outcomes should receive priority in the plan?

Which of these measures should (be included) (receive priority) in the care plan for a client who (has nursing dx, medical dx)?

When a client (has nursing dx, medical dx, manifestation) (is receiving medication), which of these (pieces of equipment, medications) should a nurse have available?

A nurse should include which of these teaching strategies when planning care for a client who has (nursing dx, med dx, developmental level)?

Which of these measures, if included in the care plan for a client who has (dx), would be most effective to (reduce, relieve) (clinical manifestation)?

The teaching plan for a client who is taking (medication or class of medication) should include which of these instructions?

When planning home care for a client who has (dx), which of these (measures) should a nurse assist the client and family to identify as the priority? Which of these referrals should a nurse make?

Which of these outcomes would be most appropriate to establish for a client who has (nursing dx)?

A nurse is planning staff assignments. Which of these clients would be the most appropriate for the nurse to assign to a nursing assistant?

A nurse should assign which of these staff members to care for (a client who has . . . , an elderly client, an anxious client)?

Which of these laboratory results would be most important for a nurse to monitor for a client who has . . . ?

Which of these nursing measures would be most effective to assist a client who has (nursing dx, medical dx) in order to achieve the outcome of . . . ?

IV. IMPLEMENTATION

Process of initiating and completing the nursing actions to accomplish the defined outcomes

A nurse should instruct a client who (has dx, is at risk for . . .) to make which of these lifestyle modifications?

A client is scheduled to start taking (medication). A nurse should teach the client to observe for side effects, which include . . .

The parents of a (. . .)-year-old child express concern to a nurse about (child's behavior). Which of these explanations (related to age/developmental level) would be most appropriate for the nurse to give the parents?

A client who has (dx) has all of these medications ordered. Which one would the nurse administer when the client complains of . . . ?

Before administering (medication, treatment) to a client, which of these (lab value, vital signs) should a nurse check?

When a client who has (dx) develops (manifestation, lab value), which of these actions should a nurse take (first, initially)?

Which of these assessments of a client who has (dx) requires immediate nursing intervention?

Which of these approaches would be most appropriate for a nurse to take when (performing a procedure) on a (age/developmental level) child?

Which of these explanations would be appropriate for a nurse to give to a client who is scheduled to have (surgery, procedure)?

A client (states, acts, experiences an unusual event) or a nurse (performs a procedure, witnesses an accident). Which of these statements would be the most appropriate for the nurse to record in the client's medical record?

A client who is scheduled for (surgery, dx procedure, treatment) says to a nurse, ". . . " Which of these responses would be most appropriate for the nurse to make?

A nurse observes a (colleague, nursing assistant) including all of these measures when (performing a procedure). Which one would require the nurse to intervene? Which of these actions is most appropriate for the nurse to take?

V. EVALUATION

Process of measuring the client's response to treatments, medications, and nursing actions and progress toward achieving defined outcomes

A client has been given instructions about (treatment, procedure, medication). Which of these statements, if made by the client, (would indicate that the client has the correct understanding of the instructions) (would indicate that the client needs FURTHER instruction)?

A client who has (dx) is (taking medication, receiving treatment). Which of these statements, if made by the client, would indicate that the (medication treatment) is having (an UNTOWARD, the desired) effect?

When a client who has a (dx) is being treated with (medication, treatment), which of these (manifestations, lab data) would indicate that the client's condition is (improving, worsening)?

A client who has (dx) is receiving (medication, treatment). Which of these responses should a nurse expect the client to have if the (medication, treatment) is achieving the desired therapeutic effect?

A client is on a (diet). Which of these meals, if selected by the client, would indicate that the client has the correct understanding of the diet plan?

A client who has (dx) is receiving (medication, treatment). Which of these (laboratory, assessment) findings should a nurse recognize as indicating that the treatment is (having the desired effect) (having an untoward effect)?

An outcome for a client who has a (dx) of (. . .) is . . . Which of these client (statements, behaviors, findings) would indicate that the interventions to meet this outcome have been (successful, UNSUCCESSFUL)?

Which of these client observations is the most reliable indicator that a client has the correct understanding of how to (give injection, follow diet, avoid side effects)?

Which of these statements is the most accurate recording of a client's response to (a medication, treatment, procedure)?

Which of these (actions, statements) of a client who has (dx) would be the best indicator of the client's acceptance of (dx, diet, death, body image change)?

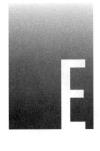

Steps for Implementing a Systematic Assessment Plan

1. Define the constructs.
2. Develop instructional objectives.
3. Write learning outcomes.
4. Outline the course content.
5. Schedule exams and due dates for other assignments.
6. Develop a grade plan based on the guidelines.
7. Identify teaching/learning activities to address course content and objectives.
8. Determine assessment tasks that are appropriate to measure the achievement of course content and objectives.
9. Determine what content and course objectives to include on each assessment task.
10. Blueprint exams and assignments to address course content and objectives.
11. Include all of the above information in the course syllabus.
12. Discuss all of the above information with the students.
13. Write exam items to address the blueprint.
14. Assemble the exams based on the blueprint specifications.
15. Review exams to verify that they meet the blueprint specifications.
16. Administer and score the exams based on the guidelines.
17. Analyze the results of the tests.
18. Assign scores to the tests.
19. Provide students with feedback regarding their achievement.
20. Offer remediation to students as needed.
21. Use item analysis to improve and bank items with their data.
22. Assign grades at the end of the semester based on a predefined grading plan.
23. Communicate the grades to students.

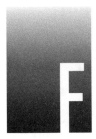

Relationship of Critical Thinking Characteristics to the Nursing Process

Critical Thinking Characteristics	Nursing Process				
	Assessment	Analysis	Planning	Implementation	Evaluation
Demonstrates sensitivity to context					
Identifies situations requiring modification	X				X
Asks relevant questions	X	X		X	X
Distinguishes subjective from objective data	X	X			X
Clarifies the meaning of information		X			X
Collects data from relevant sources	X				X
Decodes the significance of data		X			
Identifies the need for additional data	X	X			X
Delegates responsibility appropriately			X	X	
Recognizes safe practice	X	X	X	X	X
Questions assumptions					
Examines presumptions about how the world works		X			
Recognizes that there is not one normal pattern	X	X	X	X	X
Clarifies beliefs and value judgments		X			
Separates fact from fallacy		X			X
Distinguishes fact from opinion		X			X
Identifies faulty reasoning		X			X

Critical Thinking Characteristics	Nursing Process				
	Assessment	Analysis	Planning	Implementation	Evaluation
Bases inquiry on credible sources					
Analyzes data based on accurate knowledge base		✗			✗
Interprets data based on accurate knowledge base		✗			✗
Recognizes assumptions and faulty reasoning		✗			
Identifies limitations of data	✗	✗			
Evaluates evidence for accuracy and relevance		✗			✗
Discriminates between accurate and inaccurate evidence		✗			
Distinguishes between relevant and irrelevant information		✗			
Uses appropriate resources	✗	✗	✗	✗	✗
Incorporates professional, ethical, and legal standards	✗	✗	✗	✗	✗
Makes inferences based on data		✗			✗
Bases actions on accurate information			✗	✗	
Considers a variety of solutions					
Guides the collaborative process	✗	✗	✗	✗	✗
Poses solutions to unique problems			✗	✗	✗
Examines alternative solutions			✗	✗	✗
Evaluates the integrity of conclusions					✗
Develops a plan of action			✗		
Prioritizes nursing interventions			✗	✗	
Identifies the client's perception of the plan					✗
Provides scientific rationale for the plan		✗	✗		
Establishes outcomes		✗	✗		✗

Critical Thinking Characteristics	Nursing Process				
	Assessment	Analysis	Planning	Implementation	Evaluation
Pursues ongoing evaluation					
Evaluates the effect(s) of the plan from a variety of perspectives			✗		✗
Seeks objective information to evaluate the plan					✗
Analyzes new information		✗			✗
Obtains input and critique from others	✗				✗
Draws conclusions about the plan's effectiveness					✗
Develops criteria for evaluation			✗		
Revises plan based on evaluation			✗	✗	

References

Adams, B. L. (1999). Nursing education for critical thinking: An integrative review. *Journal of Nursing Education,* 38(3), 111–119.

Airasian, P. W. (1997). *Classroom assessment.* New York: McGraw-Hill.

Alfaro-LeFevre, R. (1995). *Critical thinking in nursing: A practical approach* (2nd ed.). Philadelphia: W. B. Saunders.

American Educational Research Association, American Psychological Association, & National Council on Measurement in Education. (1985). *Standards for educational and psychological testing.* Washington, D.C.: American Educational Research Association.

American Educational Research Association, American Psychological Association, & National Council on Measurement in Education. (1999). *Standards for educational and psychological testing.* Washington, D.C.: American Educational Research Association.

American Federation of Teachers, National Council on Measurement in Education, & National Education Association. (1990). *Standards for teacher competence in educational assessment of students.* Washington, D.C.: National Council on Measurement in Education.

Anastasi, A., & Urbina, S. (1997). *Psychological testing* (7th ed.). Upper Saddle River, NJ: Prentice Hall.

Angelo, T. A., & Cross, K. P. (1993). *Classroom assessment techniques: A handbook for college teachers* (2nd ed.). San Francisco: Josey-Bass.

Bandman, E. L., & Bandman, B. (1995). *Critical thinking in nursing* (2nd ed.). Norwalk, CT: Appleton and Lange.

Bloom, B. S. (Ed.), Englehart, M. D., Furst, E. J., Hill, W. H., & Krathwohl, D. R. (1956). *Taxonomy of educational objectives: The classification of educational goals.* New York: Longmans, Green and Co.

Bond, L. A. (1996). *Norm-and criterion-referenced testing.* Washington, D.C.: The Catholic University of America Department of Education. (ERIC/AE Digest Series EDO-TM-96-09).

Bower, D., Linc, L., & Denega, D. (1988). *Evaluation instruments in nursing.* New York: National League for Nursing.

Brookhart, S. M. (1999). *The art and science of classroom assessment: The missing part of pedagogy.* Washington, D.C.: The George Washington University Graduate School of Education and Human Development. (ERIC Document Reproduction Service No. ED 432 937).

Browne, M. N. (1994). *Asking the right questions: A guide to critical thinking* (5th ed.). Upper Saddle River, NJ: Prentice Hall.

Burns, N., & Grove, S. K. (1997). *The practice of nursing research* (3rd ed.). Philadelphia: W. B. Saunders.

Case, B. C. (1994). Walking around the elephant: A critical-thinking strategy for decision making. *The Journal of Continuing Education in Nursing, 25*(3), 101–109.

Chenevey, B. C. (1988). Constructing multiple-choice examinations: Item writing. *The Journal of Continuing Education in Nursing, 19*(5), 201–204.

Choudry, U. K. (1992). New nurse faculty: Core competence for role development. *Journal of Nursing Education, 31*(6), 265–272.

Cizek, G. J. (1999). *Cheating on tests: How to do it, detect it, and prevent it.* Mahwah, NJ: Lawrence Erlbaum Associates.

Clements, H., & MacDonald, J. (1966). Moral concerns in assessing pupil growth. *The National Elementary School Principal, 45,* 29–33.

Commission on Collegiate Nursing Education (CCNE). (1998). *CCNE standards for accreditation of baccalaureate and graduate nursing education programs.* Washington, D. C.: Author. [Online]. Available: http://www.aacn.nche.edu/accreditation/index.html.

Conger, M. M., & Mezza, I. (1996). Fostering critical thinking in nursing students in the clinical setting. *Nurse Educator, 21*(3), 11-15.

Davis, D. C., Dearman, C., Schwab, C., & Kitchens, E. (1992). Competencies of novice nurse educators. *Journal of Nursing Education, 31*(4), 159–164.

Dexter, P., Applegate, M., Backer, J., Claytor, K., Keffer, J., Norton, B., & Ross, B. (1997). A proposed framework for teaching and evaluating critical thinking in nursing. *Journal of Professional Nursing, 13*(3), 160–167.

DeYoung, S., & Beshore-Bliss, J. (1995). Nursing faculty—An endangered species? *Journal of Professional Nursing, 11*(2), 84–88.

Diestler, S. (1998). *Becoming a critical thinker: A user-friendly manual* (2nd ed.). Upper Saddle River, NJ: Prentice Hall.

Ebel, R. L. (1979). *Essentials of educational measurement* (3rd ed.). Englewood Cliffs, NJ: Prentice Hall.

Ennis, R. H. (1985). A logical basis for measuring critical thinking skills. *Educational Leadership, 43,* 44–48.

Facione, N. C., Facione, P. A., & Sanchez, C. A. (1994). Critical thinking disposition as a measure of competent clinical judgement: The development of the California Critical Thinking Disposition Inventory. *Journal of Nursing Education,* 33(8), 345–350.

Feingold, C., & Perlich, L. J. (1999). Teaching critical thinking through a health-promotion contract. *Nurse Educator,* 24(4), 42–44.

Fitzpatrick, M. L., & Heller, B. R. (1980). Teaching the teachers to teach. *Nursing Outlook,* 26(6), 372–373.

Ford, J. S., & Profetto-McGrath, J. (1994). A model for critical thinking within the context of curriculum as praxis. *Journal of Nursing Education,* 33(8), 341–344.

Frary, R. (1995). *How difficult should a test be?* Blacksburg, VA: Virginia Polytechnic Institute and State University. (ERIC/AE Digest series EDO-TM-95-6).

Frary, R. (1995). *More multiple-choice item writing do's and don'ts.* Blacksburg, VA: Virginia Polytechnic Institute and State University. (ERIC/AE Digest series EDO-TM-95-4).

Frisbe, D. A. (1988). Reliability of scores from teacher-made tests. *Educational Measurement: Issues and Practice,* 7(1), 25–35.

Frisbe, D. A., & Waltman, K. K. (1992). Developing a personal grading plan. *Educational Measurement: Issues and Practice,* 11(3), 35–42.

Gaberson, K. B. (1996). Test design: Putting all the pieces together. *Nurse Educator,* 21(4), 28–33.

Green, C. (2000). *Critical thinking in nursing: Case studies across the curriculum.* Upper Saddle River, NJ: Prentice Hall.

Gronlund, N. E. (1973). *Preparing criterion-referenced tests for classroom instruction.* New York: Macmillan.

Gronlund, N. E. (1993). *How to make achievement tests and assessments.* Needham Heights, MA: Allyn and Bacon.

Gronlund, N. E. (2000). *How to write and use instructional objectives* (6th ed.). Upper Saddle River, NJ: Prentice Hall.

Gullickson, A. R., & Ellwein, M. C. (1985). Post hoc analysis of teacher-made tests: The goodness-of-fit between prescription and practice. *Educational Measurement: Issues and Practice,* 4(2), 15–18.

Guskey, T. R. (1994). Making the grade: What benefits students? *Educational Leadership,* 51(10), 14–20.

Haladyna, T. M., & Downing, S. M. (1989). A taxonomy of multiple-choice item-writing rules. *Applied Measurement in Education,* 2(1), 37–50.

Haladyna, T. M. (1997). *Writing test items to evaluate higher order thinking.* Needham Heights, MA: Allyn and Bacon.

Haladyna, T. M. (1999). *A complete guide to student grading.* Needham Heights, MA: Allyn and Bacon.

Haladyna, T. M. (1999). *Developing and validating multiple-choice test items* (2nd ed.). Mahwah, NJ: Lawrence Erlbaum.

Hambleton, R. K, & Rodgers, J. H. (1995). Item bias review. *Practical Assessment, Research & Evaluation,* 4(6). [Online]. Available: http://ericae.net/pare/getvn.asp?v=4&n=6.

Hambleton, R. K., & Rodgers, J. H. (1996). *Developing an item bias review form.* [Online]. Available: http://ericae.net/ft//tsamu/biaspub2.htm.

Hertz, J. E., Yocum, C. J., & Gawel, S. H. (1999). *Linking the NCLEX-RN national licensure examination to practice: 1999 practice analysis of newly licensed registered nurses in the U.S.* Chicago: National Council of State Boards of Nursing.

Huba, M. E., & Freed, J. E. (2000). *Learning-centered assessment on college campuses: Shifting the focus from teaching to learning.* Boston: Allyn and Bacon.

Impara, J. C. (1995). *Assessment skills of counselors, principals, and teachers.* (ERIC Document Reproduction Service No. ED 387 708).

Jacobs, P. M., Ott, B., Sullivan, B., Ulrich, Y., & Short, L. (1997). An approach to defining and operationalizing critical thinking. *Journal of Nursing Education,* 36(1), 19–22.

Jenkins, P., & Turick-Gibson, T. (1999). An exercise in critical thinking using role playing. *Nurse Educator,* 24(6), 11–14.

Kataoka-Yahiro, M., & Saylor, C. (1994). A critical thinking model for nursing judgment. *Journal of Nursing Education,* 33(8), 351–356.

Kehoe, J. (1995). Writing multiple-choice test items. *Practical Assessment, Research & Evaluation,* 4(9). [Online]. Available: http://ericae.net/pare/getvn.asp?v=4&n=9.

Kehoe, J. (1995). Basic item analysis for multiple-choice tests. *Practical Assessment, Research & Evaluation,* 4(10). [Online]. Available: http://ericae.net/pare/getvn.asp?v=4&n=10.

Klisch, M. L. (1994). Guidelines for reducing bias in nursing examinations. *Nurse Educator,* 19(2), 35–39.

Koch, F. T., & Speers, A. T. (1997). It is time to move from the nursing process to critical thinking. *AORN Journal,* 66(2), 318–320.

Linn, R. L., & Gronlund, N. E. (2000). *Measurement and assessment in teaching.* Upper Saddle River, NJ: Prentice Hall.

Lyman, H. B. (1998). *Test scores and what they mean.* Boston: Allyn and Bacon.

Lynn, M. R. (1986). Determination and quantification of content validity. *Nursing Research,* 35(8), 382–385.

Mager, R. F. (1962). *Preparing instructional objectives.* Belmont, CA: Fearon Publishers.

Mastrian, K. G., & McGonigle, D. (1999). Using technology-based assignments to promote critical thinking. *Nurse Educator,* 24(1), 45–47.

McMillan, J. H. (1997). *Classroom assessment: Principles and practice for effective instruction.* Boston: Allyn and Bacon.

Mehrens, W. A., & Lehmann, I. J. (1973). *Measurement and evaluation in education and psychology*. New York: Holt, Rinehart and Winston.

Miller, M. A., & Malcolm, N. S. (1990). Critical thinking in the nursing curriculum. *Nursing & Health Care*, 11(2), 67–73.

Morrison, S., Smith, P., & Britt, R. (1996). *Critical thinking and test item writing*. Livingston, TX: Health Education Systems.

Moskal, B. M., & Leydens, J. A. (2000). Scoring rubric development: Validity and reliability. *Practical Assessment, Research & Evaluation*, 7(10). [Online]. Available: http://ericae.net./pare/getvn.asp?v=7&n=10.

National Council on Measurement in Education Ad Hoc Committee on the Development of a Code of Ethics. (1995). *Code of professional responsibilities in educational measurement*. Washington, D.C.: Author.

National Council of State Boards of Nursing. (1995). *Test plan for the National Council licensure examination for registered nurses*. Chicago: Author.

National Council of State Boards of Nursing. (1997). *Test plan for the National Council licensure examination for registered nurses*. Chicago: Author.

National Council of State Boards of Nursing. (1998). *National Council detailed test plan for the NCLEX-RN examination*. Chicago: Author.

National Council of State Boards of Nursing. (2000). *Test plan for the National Council licensure examination for registered nurses*. Chicago: Author.

National League for Nursing Accrediting Commission. (2000). *Accreditation manual 2000*. New York: Author.

National League for Nursing Accrediting Commission. (2000). *Planning for ongoing systematic evaluation and assessment of outcomes*. New York: Author.

Nitko, A. J. (1996). *Educational assessment of students* (2nd ed.). Englewood Cliffs, NJ: Prentice-Hall.

Nunnally, J. C. (1964). *Educational measurement and evaluation*. New York: McGraw-Hill.

Oermann, M. H. (1990). Psychomotor skill development. *Journal of Continuing Education in Nursing*, 21(5), 202–204.

Oermann, M. H., & Gaberson, K. B. (1990). *Evaluation and testing in nursing education*. New York: Springer.

Ory, J. C., & Ryan, K. E. (1993). *Tips for improving testing and grading*. Newbury Park, London: Sage.

O'Sullivan, P. S., Blevins-Stephens, W. L., Smith, F. M., & Vaughn-Wrobel, B. (1997). Addressing the National League for Nursing critical-thinking outcome. *Nurse Educator*, 22(1), 23–29.

Pardue, S. F. (1987). Decision-making skills and critical thinking ability among associate degree, diploma, baccalaureate, and master's prepared nurses. *Journal of Nursing Education*, 26(9), 354–361.

Paul, R. W. (1993). *Critical thinking: What every person needs to survive in a rapidly changing world* (3rd ed.). Santa Rosa, CA: Foundation for Critical Thinking.

Polit, D. F., & Hungler, B. P. (1999). *Nursing research: Principles and methods.* Philadelphia: Lippincott Williams & Wilkins.

Pond, E. F., Bradshaw, M. J., & Turner, S. L. (1991). Teaching strategies for critical thinking. *Nurse Educator*, 16(1), 18–22.

Popham, W. J. (1999). *Classroom assessment: What teachers need to know.* Boston: Allyn and Bacon.

Reilly, D. E., & Oermann, M. H. (1990). *Behavioral objectives: Evaluation in nursing* (3rd ed.). New York: National League for Nursing.

Roid, G. H., & Haladyna, T. M. (1982). *A technology for test-item writing.* New York: Academic Press.

Rubenfeld, M. G., & Scheffer, B. K. (1999). *Critical thinking in nursing* (2nd ed.). Philadelphia: Lippincott Williams & Wilkins.

Rudner, L. M. (1994). Questions to ask when evaluating tests. *Practical Assessment, Research & Evaluation, 4*(2). [Online]. Available: http://ericae.net/pare/getvn.asp?v=4&n=2.

Rudner, L. M. (1998). Item banking. *Practical Assessment, Research & Evaluation, 6*(4). [Online]. Available: http://ericae.net/pare/getvn.asp?v=6&n=4.

Schoolcraft, V. (1989). *A nuts-and-bolts approach to teaching nursing.* New York: Springer.

Slavin, R. E. (1997). *Educational Psychology* (5th ed.). Boston: Allyn and Bacon.

Smith-Stoner, M. (1999). *Critical thinking activities for nursing.* Philadelphia: Lippincott Williams & Wilkins.

Steele, D., & Wendt, A. (1999). *National Council detailed test plan for the NCLEX-RN examination.* Chicago: National Council of State Boards of Nursing.

Stiggins, R. J. (1999). Evaluating classroom assessment training in teacher education programs. *Educational Measurement: Issues and Practice*, 18(1), 23–27.

Thorndike, R. M. (1997). *Measurement and evaluation in psychology and education* (6th ed.). Upper Saddle River, NJ: Prentice Hall.

Tomey, A. M. (1999). Testing techniques: Preparing a testing blueprint from levels of course objectives. *Nurse Educator*, 24(4), 11–12.

Trice, A. D. (2000). *A handbook of classroom assessment.* New York: Longman.

Videbeck, S. L. (1997). Critical thinking: A model. *Journal of Nursing Education*, 36(1), 23–28.

Walvoord, B. E., & Anderson, V. J. (1998). *Effective grading.* San Francisco: Jossey-Bass.

Ward, A. W., & Murray-Ward, M. (1994). Guidelines for the development of item banks. *Educational Measurement: Issues and Practice*, 13(1), 34–39.

Weimer, M. (1996). *Improving your classroom teaching.* Newbury Park, CA: Sage.

Weis, P. A., & Guyton-Simmons, J. (1998). A computer simulation for teaching critical thinking skills. *Nurse Educator*, 23(2),30–33.

Westwick, C. R. (1976). Item analysis. *Journal of Nursing Education*, 15(5), 27–32.

White, N. E., Beardslee, N. O., Peters, D, & Supples, J. M. (1990). Promoting critical thinking skills. *Nurse Educator*, 15(5), 16–19.

Worthen, B. R., Borg, W. R., & White, K. (1993). *Measurement and evaluation in the schools*. White Plains, NY: Longman.

Yocum, C. J. (1997). *Job analysis newly licensed registered nurses 1996*. Chicago: National Council of State Boards of Nursing.

Yocum, C. J., & White, E, L. (1999). *1999 licensure and examination statistics*. Chicago: National Council of State Boards of Nursing.

Index

Note: **boldface** numbers indicate illustrations; italic *t* indicates a table.